Advanc

What the Honeybees Taught Me
How 10,000 Stings Improved Both My MS and My Life

MARILYN MURRAY WILLISON

"Truly fascinating! Marilyn Murray Willison continues to astonish with her thought-provoking work."

Judy Blume
Winner of over 90 Literary Awards, and a Library of Congress Living Legend

"Willison gifts us the tools to reframe our life experiences as we learn that there can be great depth and meaning from seemingly mundane events. The key, as she reveals, is to remain open and aware for the guidance that cradles us all."

David Perlmutter, MD
Author, #1 New York Times bestseller *Grain Brain,* and *Drop Acid*

"Marilyn Murray Willison, the bravest of patients, takes us on a riveting and fascinating journey into the world of thousands of stings in her miraculous alliance with honeybees to treat her multiple sclerosis."

Delia Ephron
Author of *Left on Tenth: A Second Chance at Life.*

"Willison's voice has just the right pitch to cut through the myopia that has seemed to engulf the post-pandemic world. The struggle of those with MS may never be completely fathomable to the majority of her readers, but we all need to hear what she has to teach us about this disease, which can be so difficult to treat. Her journey to honey bees is as much a journey through the wilderness of mental stress, health setbacks and at times, true breakthroughs to freedom and joy as it is an adventure into the world of beekeepers, apitherapy and of course, the bees themselves."

Dr. Tammy Horn Potter
Kentucky State Apiarist and author of *Bees in America: How the Honey Bee Shaped a Nation*

"This book is an amazing narrative on the use of bee venom, honey, propolis, bee pollen and other hive products to treat multiple sclerosis, by an MS patient who used an Apitherapist to deal with her condition

after neurologists threw away the towel. Enjoy and learn about honeybees, bravery, and Willison's beautiful life journey."

Moisés Asís, PhD, MSW, JD
Author of *Apiterapia 101 Para Todos*, and fifteen other bee-related books

"Marilyn Murray Willison's latest book is must-read. Her work is thought-provoking, informative, educational, personal, and straight from the heart. I have known her (and her books!) for over 25 years and always look forward to her sharing with us her life experiences. Travel with her through her interesting stories and be touched by her love and life. I know you will be enriched, inspired, and energized. Enjoy! "

William H. Stager, DO, MS, MPH, FAAFP, FAAMA, FAAO, FACOFP dist.
Board Certified in Family Medicine, as well as Neuromusculoskeletal Medicine and Osteopathic Manipulative Medicine Clinical Professor of Family Medicine, NSUKPCOM

"As someone with my own serious chronic illness, I appreciate Marilyn's openness and her willingness to be vulnerable as she shares her experiences. In What

the Honeybees Taught Me, she both educates and inspires. Her passion for life and learning is uplifting and sure to resonate with her readers."

Diane Chamberlain

New York Times bestselling author of *The Last House on the Street*

"A must-read book for any patient who has not yet found an effective path toward healing. Willison's book stimulates our creativity, intelligence, love, intuition, will and courage, e.g., all the things needed before one starts a new health-oriented life project."

Dr. Stefan Stangaciu (Romania)

Preventive medical practitioner with emphasis on the use of bee products, and author of four apiphyto-aromatherapy books.

"As befits an award-winning journalist, Willison's writing style effectively blends memoirs with accessible, engaging, informational text....A compelling and informative celebration of honeybees and exploration of their potential for medical treatment."

Kirkus Reviews

Medical Disclosure

ALSO BY
MARILYN MURRAY WILLISON

*BE BOLD: CULTIVATING
HEALTH AND HAPPINESS FOR
OLDER ADULTS*

*ONE WOMAN, FOUR DECADES,
EIGHT WISHES*

THE SELF-EMPOWERED WOMAN

*WHEN YOUR LIFE INCLUDES A
WHEELCHAIR*

THE SELF-CONFIDENCE TRICK

TIME ENOUGH FOR LOVE

DIARY OF A DIVORCED MOTHER

What the Honeybees Taught Me

How 10,000 Stings Improved Both My MS and My Life

Marilyn Murray Willison

For Jeanne Hunter,

whose generous heart made the bee
stings possible.

"One of my convictions is that the more you know about anything, the more interested in it you are."

Gavin Larsen
BEING A BALLERINA

"School is everywhere."

James Edward Murray
(1903-1968)

TABLE OF CONTENTS

Page

INTRODUCTION

The story of bees begins with biology, but it also tells us about ourselves.... People study bees to better understand everything from collective decision-making to addiction, architecture, and efficient public transportation. As social animals recently adapted to living in large groups, we have a lot to learn from a group of creatures who, in part at least, have been doing it successfully for millions of years.

BUZZ
Thor Hanson (1947-2018)

Today, our bodies (just like our planet) are currently under attack from chemicals, pesticides, pollution, stress, viruses, and whatever other unclassified environmental threats may cross our path. If any of those concerns raise a blip on your personalized radar screen, then my lengthy and unusual journey—which involved pain, patience, tenacity, transformation, and wonder—just might inspire you to become a fellow honeybee afficionado.

According to research, there is so much interest in the elusive and mysterious honeybee that there are already over 10,000 books in print about them on Amazon at this time. Not surprisingly, the majority of those volumes have been written by either enthusiastic and devoted beekeepers or by brilliant academic researchers.

1

My story is different. Unlike most "bee people," I never had a youthful encounter with *Apis mellifera* that later blossomed into a lifelong passion for the amazing little insects that are genetically programmed to be continuously productive. In fact, the closest I ever came to knowing anything at all about bees as a youngster was from the plastic honey-filled bear-shaped squeeze bottles that my mother regularly purchased at the local grocery store.

I enjoyed an enviably healthy childhood, and probably ingested gallons of golden sweet honey, but I did so blithely without any curiosity whatsoever regarding its origins. Then, inexplicably, practically every aspect of my life changed over time, and honeybees became very important indeed. The years had sped by, the decades had piled on top of one another, and before I knew or understood what had happened I'd somehow managed to become a wheelchair-dependent, disabled senior citizen. But as Pulitzer-prize winning writer Gail Caldwell has observed, "Watch enough decades go by, and every path has broken stones along the way."

The agent of this unfortunate development was labelled *Multiple Sclerosis*. For those of you who may not know, MS is a devastating neurological condition that is occasionally known as a "slow stroke" because of the gradual and progressive—rather than sudden—loss of physical function. There are currently close to a million Americans who have MS, and our varied symptoms can range from debilitating fatigue to lack of muscle control to visual difficulties as well as vocal challenges. MS is terrifying, and it can turn your entire life upside down.

***

This is a book about how and why I became obsessed with information regarding anything and everything that has to do with honeybees. In my quest for knowledge and better understanding, I read dozens of books, watched countless documentaries, pestered local beekeepers, and did my best to unravel one of the natural world's biggest (and sweetest) mysteries. In what became a massive—and much-needed—stroke of good luck, before I knew what had happened, I had turned into an obsessed 70-year-old Bee Geek.

In my case, by the time COVID-19 arrived in America, I was a profoundly disabled woman who had been in a wheelchair for three decades. The only functioning part of my stiff and paralyzed body that I could still move at will was my left arm. Years before, in the midst of my escalating challenges, I'd been lucky enough to meet, fall in love with, and marry an exceptionally kind, handsome and loving man, Tony, who'd had a sister-in-law with MS. He knew the drill regarding this disease, wasn't intimidated by my increasing disability, was determined to keep me smiling, and conscientiously watched over my body's gradual decline.

Then, after 20 happy years together, he died following a valiant struggle with cancer. No matter how hard I tried to be positive, during that dark time it seemed as if each lonely new day brought more and more emotional and physical challenges.

***

Years earlier, Tony and I had watched a *60 Minutes* segment that profiled an alternative health practice known as Bee Venom Therapy (BVT). At that time, honeybee venom was rumored to have a potentially positive impact on certain chronic autoimmune conditions—including MS. In spite of our best efforts, we'd never been able to locate anyone in South Florida with the skillset to safely administer BVT stings.

Then, in 2019—two years after Tony's death—Hudson Valley resident Penelope Queen gave my dear friend, Jeanne Hunter, the name of a local beekeeper who lived only a few miles from my house. I was soon able to meet the patient and experienced apitherapists Michael Szakacs and Professor Vetaley Stashenko, and things started to subtly but incrementally change for the better. Those two generous beekeepers brought with them a kind and skilled sense of possibility that gave me (for the first time in ages) a glimmer of hope that replaced the grim acceptance that had dominated my life for years. That casual but all-important introduction was when my love affair with honeybees began, and when my broken heart—as well as my disabled body—slowly began to heal.

***

Those of you who are familiar with my earlier memoirs, know only too well that my entire life has consisted of unpredictable roller-coaster highs and very scary lows. The good news is that while those unwelcomed twists of fate frequently brought me to my knees and bruised my soul, they never broke my spirit. Somehow (for the most part), as I stumbled from one crisis to another, I managed to remain a Stubborn Optimist. Against all odds, I continued to believe that **Something Wonderful Is About to Happen**.

Even during my most challenging episodes—and there have been plenty—I have always clung to the belief that I am a fortunate person who was born under a lucky star. Why would I think such a thing? Because, inevitably, some sort of compensatory twist of fate has almost always miraculously come my way after every single setback I've ever endured. Back in 2019, that blessing took the form of two middle-aged beekeepers who were determined to do whatever they could to help me feel better.

***

I wanted to write this memoir as a protracted thank you note to the driven and hard-working female insects that taught me so many unexpected and valuable life lessons. My years with the bees (and a wide variety of their byproducts) have shown me that the small can be strong, that cooperation can accomplish the astonishing, that pain frequently includes a powerful payoff, and that there is often more than one way to get what you want—as well as what you need.

I decided to write this book because I had four very personal goals; it was important for me to:

- tell the story of how honeybees affected my health and (literally) changed my life.
- remind readers that—for thousands of years and on every continent except Antarctica—honeybees have been pollinating our crops and directly contributing to humans' food supply.
- spread the word about how bee products—from bee (hive) air to honeycomb to propolis (aka Ukrainian penicillin) to bee pollen and royal jelly—can measurably improve our wellbeing.
- and, finally, introduce the concept of bee venom therapy (BVT) as a potential form of "acupuncture on steroids."

Essentially, this book is the unlikely story of how paying close attention to the honeybees—and getting a few dozen bee venom stings each week—totally altered my attitude toward (and outlook about) almost everything in my life for the better.

In light of what I experienced, I'm willing to wager that the more you appreciate and know about honeybees the more likely it is that various aspects of your own wellbeing just may gradually and mysteriously be enhanced as well. After all, honeybees have been magically and continuously making life sweeter on this planet for countless centuries.

There's a part of me that will always think of those incredibly competent little hard-working insects as Mother Nature's original feminists, and I will always be grateful to them for giving me the much-needed dual priceless gifts of hope and improved health.

The pages that follow were designed to help you imagine in what ways those miracle-working honeybees just might gradually, inexplicably, and subtly make your life better as well...

Chapter 1
The Fear Factor

Do not be afraid; our fate cannot be taken from us;
it is a gift.

INFERNO
Dante Alighieri (1265-1321)

For practically my entire life, I have been on a first-name basis with fear. And the first time I heard what sounded—to my inexperienced ears—like the irritated buzzing of several dozen honeybees that were trapped in a large glass jar from across the room, I couldn't help but wonder, *"OMG, what have I got myself into? This may be more than I had bargained for."*

***

For decades, a number of my well-meaning friends have confided that they've always considered me to be a strong woman because I have survived so many challenging life situations. While that may or may not be true, I am well aware that others may see me as strong, but I have definitely never thought of myself as someone who is brave. I've never sought out danger, longed for thrills, or participated in any obviously risky activities. And that first at-home exposure to a visiting cluster of trapped honeybees reinforced my self-image as a sporadically Stubborn Optimist who was definitely feeling frightened.

After years of dead-end efforts to learn more about the impact of honeybee venom on MS symptoms, my friends and I had finally been lucky enough to get referred to a knowledgeable local South Florida beekeeper. And that's how, on a hot and humid Saturday morning, I had my first introduction to Apitherapy—the centuries-old art and science of using bees and beehive products to improve one's health and wellbeing. It was a life-changing exposure to a tiny bit of venom from an amazing creature known as *Apis mellifera*—the honeybee.

Michael was a smiling and clean-cut 40-ish accountant who exuded a quiet aura of kindness and confidence. He was a healthy-looking man of medium build who had endured his own physical problems; years earlier he had actually been bedridden with psoriatic arthritis. Bee venom therapy (BVT) had helped restore his mobility, and he is now so physically fit that he spends his Saturday mornings refereeing high school soccer matches.

But I didn't know any of that on the morning of June 29, 2019, when I nervously waited for this stranger—a highly recommended alternative health practitioner—to ring my doorbell. After weeks of email and cellphone conversations, we'd coordinated our schedules, and the day had finally arrived when I would receive my first exposure to bee venom therapy from a live (and very annoyed) honeybee.

As I waited for Michael to arrive for our first meeting, I found myself wrestling with opposing emotions. On one hand, I was excited at the prospect of an all-natural alternative health treatment that might bring my beleaguered body some relief. But on the other hand, I was worried that the live bee stings might hurt too much for me to tolerate the pain.

***

Before my life-altering diagnosis, I had known very little about MS. Since then, I've learned that it's an extremely complicated and tricky disease that can affect each patient in a uniquely harmful way. The long list of potentially devastating symptoms can vary from loss of vision to paralysis to severe muscular pain to compromised vocal cords. Back in 1984, I had been genuinely frightened by my diagnosis, but I'd defiantly refused to accept it. For years, I had been emotionally devastated by the mere suggestion that my reliably healthy body could potentially have a progressive neurological illness. The manner in which I dealt with my deeply-buried fear was that I simply denied the likelihood that I could actually have MS. The skeptic and the Stubborn Optimist in me hoped that something—anything— other than MS was to blame for my debilitating symptoms.

In retrospect, it probably would have been wiser to have been obsessive about research and information from the very beginning of my physical problems, rather than waiting decades to finally explore what *Multiple Sclerosis* would (or could) do to my body. When I belatedly decided to arm myself with a workable background of knowledge about what MS actually is, one of the first things I learned was that our bodies have one essential nervous system with two functions: motor for movement, and sensory for feeling. Many MS patients experience numbness, particularly in their extremities, because of damage to the myelinated sheath of motor neurons and axons. While others—like me—are unable to move our limbs, but the ability to feel (especially pain) is not compromised at all.

***

For years—long before my first bee sting—I had only been able to move my left arm, but my body's ability to experience discomfort was as acute as ever. For example, if a mosquito bit my left arm, I would have no way of scratching the bite, but I could definitely feel the sting as well as the resultant itch that went along with the hungry and hostile insect's bite.

Most people are much more frightened of bees than of mosquitos, but scientific research indicates that they shouldn't be. According to the National Institutes of Health (NIH), mosquitoes—unlike bees—are dangerous because they can spread a variety of diseases, including Dengue Fever, Malaria, several forms of Encephalitis, Yellow Fever, as well as West Nile and Zika viruses. Mosquito-borne illnesses kill over a million people each year, which is why many experts consider mosquitoes to be the deadliest animal on earth.

While a bee sting delivers venom that many cultures believe has health-promoting qualities, *Culicidae* (mosquito) stings are both unproductive and hurtful. For years, conventional wisdom has proposed that mosquito bites are actually the result of maternal insects that are simply in search of blood, which is needed to feed their offspring.

***

The official name for the wide variety of potentially beneficial bee items is Apitherapeutical products, and they have been in use for centuries. The therapeutic use of bee venom has been recorded as far back as the Ebers Papyrus in 1700 B.C., and it has also been recorded in a variety of religious writings, including the Bible, the Koran, and the Veda. The practice of administering bee stings was widely used in ancient Egypt, Greece, and China long before it became accepted in more recent times. Two famous historical figures who relied on bee venom therapy include Charlemagne (748-814) for gout, as well as Ivan IV the Terrible (1530-1584) for joint pain.

Unlike mosquitos, bees are respected in a variety of cultures, the art and science of beekeeping is an accepted academic program throughout several countries in Eastern Europe, as well as in Australia, Canada, China, Japan, and New Zealand. Here in the U.S. (particularly at both Cornell and UC Davis), we are finally beginning to look beyond the sometimes scary sting and acknowledge all the positive contributions that bees make to humans and to our planet's ecosystem. Instead of being irrationally afraid of bees, we are finally learning how to be grateful for all the gifts they give us.

***

Obviously, being a "triplegic" for several decades had been exceptionally challenging—both physically and emotionally. For years, I'd done my very best to be a Stubborn Optimist who avoided complaining, but I'd reached the point where I was totally fed up with the distasteful life-altering ramifications of living with MS. By 2019—35 years after my original diagnosis—I was willing to grab at any straw (even a painful or questionable one) that might bring even a modicum of improvement my way.

One of the hardest things about receiving an MS diagnosis is when a neurologist informs you that your illness is irreversible, and that your disease *might* be managed, but it will *never* be cured. According to conventional AMA wisdom, when it comes to MS, the patient's condition will be slightly worse each new day than it had been the day before. For someone who tends to be as Pollyanna-ish as I am, it was devastating to be told that my health (which essentially meant every single aspect of my existence) would never ever improve. So, yes, on that sweltering Saturday morning, I was more than willing to try anything, even if it included being stung by trapped and annoyed honeybees.

The open-minded and Stubborn Optimist part of me, however, couldn't help but recoil when Michael, the kind and clean-cut beekeeper who had been recruited by a fellow apitherapist in upstate New York, walked into my living room with a one-gallon glass jar. It held an empty cardboard paper towel roll that had been smeared with a bit of honey, as well as two dozen agitated and loudly buzzing honeybees. I don't mind admitting that I instantaneously felt frightened.

After our slightly awkward introductory pleasantries, Michael—in a calm and quiet voice—explained that he would use long stainless-steel tweezers to capture a single worker bee by her thorax, and then remove her from her portable and temporary home. He planned to test my allergic potential by giving me a single sting, and then watch to see how my body reacted; he kept a brand new EpiPen kit within arm's reach. As frightened as I was of the honeybees, however, just one look at the intimidating size of the large EpiPen needle was enough to make me want to align myself with *Apis mellifera* rather than with Big Pharma.

As I warily eyed Michael's large jar of irritated honeybees, I knew that my sensory nerves would soon be under attack. This was going to be one of those rare and bizarre times in my life that would require me to be both strong and brave.

Seated in my recliner, which is where I spend a about 90% of my time these days, I began to silently question the wisdom of making such an unorthodox commitment. *Would I experience anaphylactic shock? Why hadn't I taken the time to find–and talk to–someone else with MS who had already experienced "bee healing" before starting on this unconventional journey? And just how painful and prolonged would this honeybee "alternative healing process" be?*

***

The use of bee venom therapy (BVT) is closely connected to the traditional Chinese medical practice of acupuncture. The concept is that we all have a form of vital energy known as *Qi* (pronounced "chee") that gives us our energy, and protects us from illnesses. The *Qi* flows through 14 different pathways in our body known as meridians, which provide nourishment (i.e. energy) to our cells, glands, muscles, organs, and tissues. Acupuncture, which has been in use for over 3,000 years, is believed to eliminate blockages of *Qi* so that the body and immune system can function as they are meant to. As Michael's recovery illustrated, the application of bee stings on those specific acupuncture points or meridians can help make this possible.

Lots of people in the alternative healing arts movement feel that honeybee stings can be an all-natural form of insect-assisted acupuncture. In China, acupuncture is believed to have begun around the year 100 BC, while in Korea and Japan (thanks to medical missionaries) it arrived about 500 years later. The French were the first Europeans to embrace the use of thin needles to stimulate the body's healing abilities, but it wasn't really welcomed in the U.S.—as well as several other Western countries—until the 20th century.

One thing that is not common knowledge—unless you are a fellow bee geek like me—is that a worker bee usually only lives for about six weeks. And to add to her shortened lifespan, she is only able to sting (a person, a hive invader, a predator, etc.) once because after she loses her stinger she will die. Oddly enough, a bee loses her stinging apparatus only if she stings a mammal. Worker bees can sting an impermeable surface, another insect, or crustacea (i.e., a creature with an exoskeleton) without dying in the process.

The good news is that I didn't go into anaphylactic shock or have a bad reaction, so the scary EpiPen and its large needle stayed in its packaging. The bad news is that the worker bee's single (suicidal) sting immediately brought tears to my eyes. A honeybee's stinger is only about 1/16th of an inch long, but when it punctures your skin—depending on which acupuncture point or specific body spot is being treated—it can feel like either a thumbtack assault or as if someone with a hammer had just slammed a two-inch metal nail into your flesh. For the record, some of the most painful and sensitive spots include the head (ears, lips, neck, scalp, etc.), either side of the spinal column, the fingers, as well as the toes.

BVT afficionados insist that—to mentally offset the discomfort—it helps to remember that (and be grateful for) the many positive features that accompany getting stung by honeybees. For starters, while the pain of a bee sting is sharp, it is also short-lived—it rarely hurts for more than just a few minutes. A mosquito bite, on the other hand, can itch for days. Also, bee venom, which is anti-bacterial, anti-inflammatory, and anti-viral, can work to gradually kickstart and strengthen your own body's immune system no matter where you get stung.

***

That first sting on my lower arm left me with a small red spot, and the sense of a circularly spreading slightly itchy sensation. Michael explained that those were "normal" side-effects of a bee sting. In other words, it looked as if I would be a perfect candidate to experience the potential benefits of BVT stings.

Since I hadn't shown any signs of being allergic, Michael suggested that I have three more stings to get the honeybees' slow-motion healing process underway. My generous friend, Jeanne, was bankrolling this experimental process, and she had come to my home before Michael arrived in order to watch the procedure. In what would become a weekly sting-session routine, Jeanne held my left hand while I pretended to be brave. I wiped away the few tears that had accompanied the first sting, considered my paralyzed body's limited health options, smiled at Jeanne and Michael, and said, *"Well, OK, let's get this unconventional honeybee venom experience underway."*

WHAT THE HONEYBEES TAUGHT ME

- The phrase *"When the student is ready the teacher will appear"* has a conflicted origin. Some people credit Buddha, while others claim that it originated with the Theosophist movement, which began in 1875, and still carries on to this day. Whatever its origins, that observation definitely applied to my fond introduction to *Apis mellifera*. It's a shame that I had to wait for over six decades to understand how amazing these little insects are, but I hope that my "late bloomer" status will more than make up for my tardy beginning.

- Like many Baby Boomers, I grew up believing that "new and improved" really meant "new and improved" products; I eventually understood that what it really meant was simply "different." Eventually, however, I learned that instead of always chasing "new," it was far more satisfying to embrace natural rather than "new" (i.e., artificial or chemical) ways of promoting good health.

- Many accepted avenues of healing used during ancient eras have survived and grown in popularity to this day. Ancient Chinese and Egyptian cures (like acupuncture and the use of bee venom) remain quietly relevant to this day.

- As anyone who has ever been told *"There is no cure"* knows, desperate times often call for equally desperate measures. When hope has faded from the horizon, and you feel as if you have nothing to lose, thinking outside the box becomes more rational and routine.

- Every payoff comes with a price tag, and the possibility of improved health is well worth the temporary pain of a honeybee sting.
- Eleanor Roosevelt (1884-1962) was right when she said *"You gain strength, courage, and confidence by every experience in which you really stop to look fear in the face.... You must do the thing you think you cannot do."*

Chapter 2
Home Sweet Home

We shape our dwellings, and afterwards our dwellings shape us.

Winston Churchill (1874-1965)

I often thought of Michael's large bee transport jar as the last "home" those selfless little worker bees—who were scheduled to sting me each week—would ever have. I soon learned that the way they arrived at my house was (as are most honeybee happenings) effective, selfless, and unique.

Michael's full-time job—his MBA is from Scotland's University of Edinburgh—is as an accountant. But he loves being both a beekeeper and an apitherapist. He recently told me that he had been stunned to learn that several members of his professional beekeeping organization had retired, and given away their hives. Shaking his head in disbelief, he confided, *"I can't imagine ever living without my beehives. Even if I no longer had a yard where I could keep them, I'd find some way to have the bees still be a part of my life."* Obviously, for Michael, honeybees are more than a hobby; they are one of Mother Nature's miracles.

On his lunch hour every Thursday, Michael would drive to my home for what soon became a joint "sting session." My fun-loving 88-year-old British friend, Jeanne, would always be the first to arrive, and each week she would bring a freshly-baked treat. Some Thursdays she would bring brownies, or a Linzer Torte, or cookies, or (Michael's favorite) a rum cake.

After several weeks of receiving stings, my curiosity got the better of me, and I asked Michael how he had the time to gather all the honeybees into his jar before driving to my house.

"I'll let you in on a little secret," he told me. *"On Wednesday night, I place some honey and a bit of cardboard in my empty jar, leave the lid off, and place it horizontally near the entrance to one of my three hives. In the morning, before I go to work, I retrieve the jar—which usually has several dozen older foraging worker bees socializing inside—and I put the lid (which has airholes in it) back on the jar. I then put it in my car, which I park in the shade, and at noon I bring them and my set of tweezers to your house for our weekly sting session."*

With each passing Thursday, Michael began to gradually apply a few more stings. What had begun as four, soon turned into six, then became eight, and eventually the number of stings slowly continued to increase into double-digit territory. Jeanne would hold my hand, my remarkable much-cherished caregiver, Ramon, would apply icepacks in order to partially numb the areas where Michael's bees would sting me, and I would continue to try to be brave. Some stings didn't really hurt at all, others would feel like an amped-up mosquito bite, some would make me grimace or grit my teeth, and a few would literally make me cry.

At first, when I was only getting a couple of stings, Michael's visit—from start to finish—could be as short as fifteen to twenty minutes, but as the number of our stings increased, so did the time we spent together. During his sessions, there would be lots of conversation and laughter, and we'd learn about his parents, who had immigrated from Hungary. It's one of several Eastern European countries where the bee culture is both strong and respected. There are even residential clinics in Russia that exclusively treat MS patients with aggressive doses of BVT.

Before we knew it, our unusual little international "gang of four" had turned my cozy home into a mini once-a-week apitherapy clinic. Jeanne, who had grown up in London, suffered from painful rheumatoid arthritis in her hands. She had visited several doctors, but her twisted arthritic fingers continued to be a problematic source of concern. The medications she'd been prescribed had not stopped the pain, and her stiff fingers were becoming more and more misshapen. Her thumb had become so inflamed that the throbbing arthritis pain would wake her in the middle of the night. She had read that a number of people with her condition had been helped by BVT, so she asked Michael if she could give it a try as well.

Michael suggested that a milder form of stings—called micro-tapping—might be beneficial. In this technique, instead of placing a live honeybee on the area in question, the apitherapist first removes the stinger from the bee, and then uses it to "tap" the area, which gently delivers a small amount of venom. I'm happy to report that—with no medication—after one year of help from the honeybees, Jeanne's fingers had visibly straightened, and she no longer had to cope with a sleep-disrupting throbbing thumb.

As a young child in the mountainous area of Guatemala, Ramon had been raised by a grandmother who kept honeybees. After watching several of our sessions, he asked Michael if he could have a few stings each week just to keep him healthy the way his *Abuela* had always been. With time, both Jeanne and Ramon—as well as a rotating roster of friends who noticed that I seemed to be looking better and feeling healthier—joined our Thursday lunchtime bee sting bandwagon.

***

Perhaps my concern about Michael's bees and their final portable "home" was triggered by my own issues about being continually uprooted throughout my entire life. It's no secret that I've always envied those lucky people who've enjoyed the soothing privilege of knowing that they have a permanent home base. In my imagination, nothing could be more emotionally satisfying than being able to return to a specific place—an actual structure—that would serve as a touchstone for life's treasured moments with cherished loved ones.

When I first heard Kenny Loggins' 1977 hit *Celebrate Me Home* (which perfectly captures the priceless sense of being able to go back to your very own personal place of safety and solace for the holidays), I was sure that the song had been written especially for me. The idea of (regardless of your age) being able to "return home" to loved ones and a specific place that's overflowing with memories has always seemed to me like the ultimate emotional luxury.

Due to my father's career, however, during my childhood our little three-person nuclear family was continually "relocated" or "transferred." As a result, by the time I graduated from UCLA, I had attended almost a dozen different schools in a variety of different states and towns. The bottom line is that I never had the comfort or luxury of living in a long-term much-loved home until I was a grown woman, and the over-scheduled stressed-out mother of two young sons. (The next chapter will introduce you to that cherished "Pretty White Up-and-Down House.")

During the past few years, I think many of us have learned first-hand that few aspects of life are as important as where and how and with whom we live. Whether your home is a high-rise penthouse, a mountain cabin, a waterfront mansion, a double-wide trailer, or a rented walk-up studio apartment, one truth remains: Everyone needs a place of personal refuge and retreat.

As we (painfully) experienced during the COVID-19 pandemic, few items have the ability to affect us as permanently and profoundly as what we call "home." During our 2020 lockdown episodes, it became abundantly clear that our domestic situation—whatever it happens be—can have serious emotional, physical, and psychological effects on our well-being.

***

Studying honeybee life taught me that even tiny insects can be both particular and protective when it comes to maintaining the various aspects of their home turf. Honeybees are particularly selective about who can stay, who must leave, and every single aspect of their chosen home is given the highest priority. And according to apiologists (bee experts), these little creatures—who only weigh 0.0053 of an ounce—have been exhibiting the same attention to detail regarding their home environment—at different spots around the globe—for millions of years.

A few years before the pandemic arrived, I began paying close attention to the undeniable brilliance of honeybees, and I discovered that—today—there are about two and a half million beehives in the U.S. This sounds like a lot, until you learn that back in the 1940s there were over six million. Interestingly, as the bee population has declined, the human population has increased. According to official Census records, in 1945, there were 139 million people who lived in the U.S., while in 2010 that number had grown to 331 million.

As I began to immerse myself in the mysteries of the *Apis mellifera* world, I suddenly noticed that—practically anywhere on the globe—these amazing little creatures seemed able to always enthusiastically adapt to whatever their version of a honeybee's haven might be. (Academics and entomologists distinguish between "nest," which signifies where bee colonies have established their own homes, and "hive," which describes a man-made structure that houses an extended honeybee family.)

Throughout the ages, honeybees have managed to adapt to an amazing geographical variety of domiciles, but they always showed a consistent level of attention to detail regardless of where—or what—they called home. Whether it was inside a tree trunk, on a desert hillside, attached to a cliff, hidden inside a cave, or even clinging to an imposing rock formation, honeybees have instinctively managed to reassemble all the essential moving parts of an orderly, antiseptic, well-functioning, and cooperative lifestyle.

Centuries ago, back when bees randomly nested in completely natural settings, the humans who sought to steal their stored honey had to destroy whatever primitive structure contained the honeycomb. Sadly, this meant that most of the annoyed bees that tried to protect their home and their honey would be either injured or killed in the process. Then, around 2,000 years ago, legend has it that honey hunters in Ireland, created small structures of braided grass or hay that became known as "skeps." The name comes from a Norse word, *skeppa*, which literally means "basket." These oval-shaped bottomless hollow "bee houses" were placed large end down, and the sides were plastered with mud and dung.

Those primitive man-made "bee houses" were the hunters' first attempt to gain nearby access to honeycomb so they wouldn't have to travel to the distant spots where bees had built their own type of nest. The honeybees—laden with nectar, pollen, and propolis—could easily enter the skep via an opening near the base. After the Middle Ages, later versions of these structures often included coils of straw that were sewn together using bits of briar, or leather strips; sometimes even cow horns were used to give the skep more stability and strength.

These early raw-material precursors to modern wooden hives usually had a single good-sized entrance at the bottom. Together, the colony "manufactured" the necessary honeycomb for both brood and honey, which rested against the skep's side. Unfortunately—just as with the bee-constructed nests—to retrieve the honey harvest, many of the bees (as well as their briar, grass, and leather man-made sanctuaries) were sacrificed in the process. That destructive form of honey gathering meant that many months would pass before any remaining bees could restore their hive and provide more honey. Essentially, though the local skep was more convenient for honey gatherers, those original hives and their occupants still usually met a disastrous fate.

By the 1700s, newer versions of skeps were often built with removable wooden (or sometimes even glass) tops. This meant that bees could build their honeycomb within a "home" that wouldn't have to be systematically demolished by the honey harvesters. These newer skeps were much more profitable to 18th Century honey-hunting beekeepers than the original ones that had been completely constructed from grass and other weaker materials.

Historically, skeps were considered to be the perfect symbol of cooperation, hard work, and stability. In 1779, Continental Currency was printed to included an image of a thirteen-layered skep, which was designed to represent the interdependency of the emerging colonies.

***

Humans have used wood—specifically logs—for their dwellings as far back as the Bronze Age, which was about 3,500 years ago. The log cabins that we typically think of as the first American wooden homes were considered to have been built in the 1600s by a Swedish colony of settlers near the Delaware river. Later, French, German, Scandinavian, and Ukrainian immigrants—who came from lands with tall straight tree trunks—helped British settlers learn how to effectively construct log cabins, which were not a familiar type of home construction for the pilgrims of that time.

Wooden domestic beehives (which replaced skeps) were first designed around the late 1700s, and by the 19th century they had become standardized, and began to be manufactured in large numbers. Today, the most commonly-used wooden beehive design is known as the Langstroth, which is named for its creator, the American inventor Reverend Lorenzo Lorraine Langstroth (1810-1895). He lived in Oxford, Ohio, and began keeping honeybees as a way to combat his chronic depression. The Reverend patented his design in 1852, and since that time it has become the standard hive style for many of the world's amateur and professional beekeepers alike, primarily because of the ease with which honeycomb can be harvested.

But the Presbyterian minister—who died at his church's pulpit right before delivering a Sunday sermon—was not actually the first beekeeper to invent the modern hive structure that became named after him.

Long before Langstroth received a patent for his wooden beehive design, a brilliant but relatively overshadowed Ukrainian named Peter Prokopovych (1775-1850), is believed to have created the very first wooden movable hive. He developed—on his own— a humane method to retrieve honey with a minimum of disturbance or damage to either the honeybees or to their homes. Because of this then-revolutionary development, he is now considered to be the Father of Commercial Beekeeping. His Eastern European hive, which made it possible to harmlessly (for both humans and insects) harvest honey, appeared on the scene three full decades before Langstroth's.

Thanks to Prokopovych's research, beekeepers were finally able to routinely (and safely) inspect and monitor the health and well-being of their bee colonies. He also established a Ukrainian beekeeping school that accepted students, was in operation for over 53 years, and graduated more than 700 qualified expert beekeepers. As a brilliant and devoted beekeeper himself, he personally owned well over 6,000 colonies.

*　*　*

In today's America, our homes are usually built with wood or bricks, and sealed with plasterboard. For honeybees, the standard modern beehive is frequently made of red cedar, and follows a distinct pattern of evenly-spaced hanging (usually eight or ten) parallel frames. Wax (or sometimes plastic) structures form the foundation of the hexagonal framework that worker bees use to construct the honeycomb. These hanging frames are then spaced far enough apart—about 5/8 of an inch—for the bees to maneuver, and to prevent the honeycombs from adhering to each other. The frames need to have a specific amount of open maneuverable "bee space" because if the area between frames is narrower than one-quarter inch, the bees will fill it with a substance called propolis (which is discussed in a later chapter), but if the bee space is too large they will fill it with excess honeycomb. When the properly-positioned hanging frames are finally loaded with honey, each hive can weigh as much as 50 pounds.

For that reason, beekeepers don't just use any ordinary wooden box. Because of the weight involved the four corners of a wooden hive should be dovetailed together, and closed with box carpenters glue and nails. Otherwise, the weight of full honeycombs can damage a poorly-assembled wooden hive. If you see boxes stacked on top of one another, the one on the bottom will usually be the nursery, while the next box will be reserved for honey and beebread storage.

I found it fascinating that—throughout history—a honeybee's hive (or nest) has traditionally been much more than just a residence or a honey-storage facility. No matter where in the world it may be—Chile, China, Denmark, New Zealand, or Turkey—there are certain domestic *Apis mellifera* population components that remain the same. These include a small number of drones, a handful of potential new Queens, the current reigning Queen Bee (who lays close to an astonishing 2,000 eggs each and every day of her six-year long lifespan), and as many as 60,000 female worker bees who rarely stop performing an amazing variety of essential jobs. For those short-lived worker bees—they usually only live for four to six weeks—the hive is an antiseptic, multi-faceted refuge that contains absolutely everything the entire multi-generational community needs, both individually and as a group.

In between flashbacks of the beautiful suburban colonial home that had too-briefly been mine, I began to think of those familiar-looking painted wooden hive boxes as finely-tuned and fully-functioning honey factories. But, in fact, honeybee hives also serve as a career-development center, a comfortable climate-controlled environment, a construction site, a food-processing factory, an information hub, a maternity ward, a refueling station, a rest stop after a hard day's work, a safe haven from predators, as well as a round-the-clock Cathedral.

We humans may be inching towards that sort of layered home-based society as well. In the past, everything from villages, to suburbia, and even high-rise condos, were referred to as "bedroom communities" because home used to primarily be a place to rest and recharge our batteries. In today's world, however. we have begun to borrow the concept of an all-inclusive multi-faceted lifestyle from the bee community, and now we also use our once-tranquil homes for a wide variety of "professional" activities. Thanks to the internet, our homes are no longer primarily comprised of bedrooms, bathrooms, and a kitchen; they have become an efficient command center for the ever-evolving list of things—artistic endeavors, exercise, shopping, working remotely—that we humans need or want to do.

***

Essentially, a honeybee hive can be viewed as a small female-dominated perpetually-active mini-castle that has a Queen but no King. The diligent productivity that takes place inside each hive is conducted by thousands of female "daughters" who look after their Queen Bee mother by keeping her groomed, hydrated, protected, warm, and well-fed. Without the worker bees' continual care and concern, the Queen would almost surely either starve or freeze to death because her one and only life skill is continually laying lots and lots of eggs. To ensure the wellbeing of all the hive inhabitants, her distaff army of thousands of female caregivers literally keep her alive and well until her unparalleled egg-laying ability atrophies.

***

Back in 1991, long before honeybees were a part of my consciousness, my wheelchair and I moved into a little house in West Palm Beach, Florida. The year before, both my legs had simply stopped working, and I was no longer able to stand or walk. As a result, I was trying my best to dilute my anxiety about what the future might hold, eliminate the tsunami of depression that had been become my constant companion, and figure out how to adapt to a whole new (terrifying) way of life.

Both my teenage sons were attending schools in Oregon, where their father lived, and I'd moved back to the States after living in London for five years. While there, my health had steadily declined to the point where I could no longer spontaneously travel to exotic locales for my once-popular exclusive celebrity interviews and profiles. Essentially, MS had robbed me of my cherished career as an international journalist—one that I'd worked so very hard to create.

The familiar sense of undeserved loss that the disease had brought my way was eerily reminiscent of the sadness and disappointment I'd felt as an often uprooted young girl. I had wept angry tears each time those childhood "relocations" had forced me to (yet again) say painful goodbyes to people and places I'd hoped would have been permanent fixtures in my life. Decades later (like a pouty and petulant spoiled child) I had become a disabled, resentful, unemployed wheelchair-bound adult who continually struggled to escape a pointless "It's just not fair" mindset.

***

But eventually, with the passage of several challenging and lonely years, I found a number of creative ways to recalibrate my counterproductive "Poor me" attitude. It took a long time, but I gradually managed to construct a pleasant, if not problem-free, different, and disabled life for myself. In full Stubborn Optimist mode, I bought a cozy, little bungalow that needed lots of attention, and eventually it became my personalized version of an all-purpose paralyzed-human hive. Like the honeybees, I worked continually to fix whatever went wrong, maintain what was right, and establish a disability-adapted customized daily routine. I wanted to turn my small South Florida home into a welcoming hive of neurologically challenged yet productive activity, as well as one of emotional renewal.

I used my limited budget to hire workers who could make the necessary changes so that my modest home would be as accessible and handicap friendly as possible. Since I could no longer drive, I learned to rely on others who could. My fingers could no longer type, but I was able to slowly dictate the book reviews, chapters, letters, and syndicated columns that allowed me to remain productive in spite of how painful my body might feel or how uncooperative my limbs might be.

***

Back in 1976, when I was in the midst of a scary divorce and worried about losing my cherished home, I stitched a beautiful "Home Sweet Home" needlepoint canvas. The colorful yarn and the different styles of stitching gave me a much-needed non-chemical form of tranquilizer to calm my frazzled nerves. Today, decades later, it still hangs in a prominent spot in my bedroom.

Unlike the honeybees, I am no longer able to move about with ease and agility to explore the world—miles at a time—outside my front door, but that's okay. The little bungalow that has become my own customized nest, and which I've grown to cherish after all these years, shelters and nourishes me no matter what else is happening during these bizarre times. And it does so, in part, thanks to the ever-growing and eclectic collection of the much-loved decorative items that it holds within its increasingly crowded walls.

***

In the natural world, the *Apis mellifera's* home—whether a nest or a hive—is sweet because of the freshly accumulated inside rows of precious golden honeycomb. And thanks to the treasured memories and items I've surrounded myself with, my small cottage has sheltered me, my wheelchair, and my determination to somehow create a much brighter future. If my little home had a name plaque, it would be "This is where Stubborn Optimism lives."

Wherever they are in the world, honeybees live an active life of self-generated productivity and near-perpetual motion. Their remarkable microscopic internal GPS systems allow them to return to the correct hive, no matter how many identical wooden boxes they might happen to see. The magnetic pull of life's roots has a power that cannot be diminished or forgotten by either the hard-working honeybees or by a lucky home-loving Stubborn Optimist like me.

My once-athletic body may be paralyzed today, but I like to think that the always-active honeybees and the unmoving me still have something very important in common: We are both lucky enough to enjoy the immeasurable blessings of a deeply cared for domicile that is much more than just our home. Where we live—whether it's an Edwardian flat in central London, a tiny stucco house in South Florida, or even a cedar, cypress, or pine wooden hive—is a uniquely clear and cherished reflection of what we love, who we are, as well as how we choose to live.

WHAT THE HONEYBEES TAUGHT ME
- When I was a schoolgirl, I wish I had known that Albert Einstein (1879-1921) had observed, *"Life is*

like riding a bicycle. To keep your balance you must keep moving." It took me a long time to understand that being uprooted and being forced to move isn't the worst of all possible fates.

- It's wise to pay attention to, invest in, and improve your own environment as much as possible—no matter where or what it might happen to be.
- Samuel Johnson (1709-1784) wisely wrote that "*To be happy at home is the ultimate result of all ambition.*"
- There is something inspiring about the fact that, like turtles, honeybees instinctively know how to (literally) take their home with them wherever they happen to go.
- In 1823, the American actor John Howard Payne (1791-1852) wisely wrote, "*Be it ever so humble, there's no place like home.*" It was part of his wildly popular song *Home Sweet Home*, and that phrase has become an accepted part of American culture.
- The Bishop of Geneva, St. François de Salle (1567-1622) shared the advice, *Fleuris là où tu es planté.* Almost 400 years later, the popular and whimsical artist Mary Englebreit made that quote, "Bloom where you are planted," a popular home-based motto throughout relocation-accustomed America.

Chapter 3
My Pretty White Up-And-Down House

The home is a sacred place where you can communicate with the four elements of the universe: earth, water, air and fire.

LIKE WATER FOR CHOCOLATE,
Laura Esquivel

Honeybees are obsessively "house proud." With good reason and with exacting standards, they appear to be pre-programed at birth to care passionately about every aspect of their home—no matter where (or what) it happens to be. Whether insect or human, being emotionally connected to where we live is one of several worthwhile traits that *Homo sapiens* and *Apis mellifera* unself-consciously share.

***

Ever since I moved to South Florida, I've heard countless stories about people's "other home." For example, my friend, Sue, owns a pretty house with an enviable outdoor orchid garden on Singer Island. But she frequently speaks nostalgically about the five-acre, six-stable "farmette" in Illinois, where she lived years ago with her big dogs and her much-loved horses.

My neighbor, Andi, fondly remembers a Tudor Place apartment in Manhattan that she used to own before she moved to West Palm Beach. It looked out onto several private parks and was only a short stroll away from the United Nations headquarters.

And my BVT buddy, Jeanne, now lives in a stunning high-rise waterfront condo with expansive ocean views. But "home" for her will always be the historic Hudson Valley estate that was originally built for officers of King George's army who were fighting in the Revolutionary War.

Thoughts of what my life was like before I moved to Florida, invariably lead to happy memories of a lovely Southern California house where I lived for eleven years during the 1970s and 1980s. Unfortunately, the property's two-story colonial home—as well as the roomy hillside garden—had (what today I would label "wheelchair-hostile") steps and stairs everywhere.

I'm sorry to say that by now it's been almost 40 years since I used those up-and-down stairways to get to the basement, to the bedrooms, or to the plants and trees that populated the backyard. My life changed when—during the 1984 Los Angeles Summer Olympics, and at the insistence of a concerned friend—I took time off from my volunteer post with the British Equestrian Team for an appointment with a neurologist. After a "simple" outpatient bone-spur procedure on two toes the month before (it was Bastille Day July 14th), my legs had still not returned to normal function (i.e., walk or move) the way they should have.

After a cursory physical examination, the doctor watched me try to balance on one leg and then quickly walk up and down his office hallway. He then he asked me if I had double vision (*No*), high cholesterol (*No*), pain (*No*), or numbness (*Yes*). He cleared his throat, said that to him it looked like MS, and advised me to "*Go home, get your affairs in order, and try to continue with your normal activities and your usual life for as long as you can.*"

At that point, the way I lived was far too demanding for me to have even considered a life dominated by a "chronic progressive neurological disease." Both at home and at the *Los Angeles Times* building, every hour of my time was scheduled. Now that I have become honeybee obsessed, I realize that I had structured the perfect hyper-productive worker bee scenario, and I was (to paraphrase the words of Edna St. Vincent Millay (1892-1950)) "*burning my candle at both ends.*"

Add to the already busy mix of activities, the fact that my life already included two lively adolescents, my full-time position as Health and Fitness Editor, plus a career as a freelance book reviewer for a variety of publications that included the *Wall Street Journal*, the *Seattle Times*, the *Denver Post*, and several other large metropolitan daily newspapers.

On weekends, the boys and I were usually at the stables most Saturdays, and there were also regular Wednesday evening trips to the ice rink.

Together, we also often took impromptu jogs to the local Baskin Robbins ice cream shop, which was exactly 1.4 miles from our front door.

Additionally, there was always some distracting event going on at home—glamorous activities like appliance repairs, bill paying, electrical problems, and leaky roof issues—that demanded stressful chunks of my energy, my money, my stretched-thin problem-solving skills, and my time.

***

Returning to the afternoon of that disastrous and heartbreaking diagnosis, I reacted to the doctor's unwelcome diagnosis with a mix of stunned disbelief and sheer terror. Alone in my car, I drove through Laurel Canyon, and cried all the way home. Simultaneously, I made up my mind that (Miss "doesn't smoke, doesn't do drugs, watches her diet, and is physically active" Health and Fitness Editor) I couldn't possibly have MS. I promised myself to avoid sharing the doctor's diagnosis and scary prognosis with my sons until I absolutely had to.

As Health and Fitness Editor, I'd had the good fortune to work with both Nathan Pritiken and Norman Cousins, who had each shared with me their belief that all medications have a toxic component, and that it was wise to avoid pharmaceuticals whenever possible. During that broken-hearted tearful drive home, I remembered their advice, and vowed to find a healthy non-toxic alternative approach to "fix" whatever was causing my problematic balance, control, and strength symptoms. And essentially—almost four decades later—that is exactly what I'm still doing.

I've relied on a wheelchair—and on the assistance of strong able-bodied helpers—instead of my own legs to get my increasingly uncooperative body from one place to another ever since 1990. That means it's been about 12,000 days (or a quarter of a million hours, but who's counting?) since I've been able to go up-and-down anything other than an elevator or a ramp.

***

When I lived on that quarter-acre plot of land in Southern California, I didn't know that honeybees often fly as far as three miles away from their hive when they are foraging for nectar. Obviously, both my fruit and flower gardens held plenty of near-by nectar for all the task-oriented bees in our suburban neighborhood. Decades later, I learned that when it came to flowers, bees are particularly fond of Calendula (which can grow all year long, and is a beautiful shade of blue), Lavender (a flower that blooms all Summer long, and is popular with all the pollinators), as well as Dandelion (this is popular with bees even though it doesn't have four of the amino acids that they need to stay healthy, which is why beekeepers and Master Gardeners regard those puffy white flowers as a "snack food item" for honeybees).

Apis mellifera are especially attracted to sweet-smelling blossoms, and they seem to prefer flowers that are blue, white, or yellow. According to experts, bees are drawn to blossoms that include a blue-violet hue because they produce a larger amount of nectar than flowers of other, darker colors. Honeybees like herbs (such as Rosemary and Oregano), and they are also fond of low-lying Mint, which grew in abundance throughout my crowded hillside backyard garden.

***

As I learned more and more about how diligently honeybees maintain their nests and their hives, I reflected about why that long-ago pretty white up-and-down house continues to still mean so much to me: Maybe it's because I'd never before been able to live in any one house for such a long time.

Ever since I left California, I've lived in several different homes, but I've always kept a framed snapshot of that beautiful two-story house on my desk. Today, all it takes is a quick glance at that photo to remind me that once upon a time there were endless hectic days and joyful nights when my body worked perfectly, and my young life overflowed with endless possibilities.

I remember that time as one in which I was chronically rushed, continually stressed, very busy, and assaulted by seemingly endless activities. Those years reflected a demanding but fun-filled lifestyle that was very (very) different from the way I live today. During that time—perhaps like the Queen Bee who stage manages her active and diverse offspring—I felt responsible for the wellbeing of my family members, my friends, my colleagues, and everyone else who was part of my warp-speed emotional orbit.

***

After that original frightening MS diagnosis in 1984, I immediately made a number of lifestyle changes. I upgraded my diet, added major nutritional supplementation, enrolled in yoga classes, and began a series of regular chiropractic manipulation appointments. As if by magic, within six months, all my "bizarre" symptoms had essentially disappeared. Six months after that positive development, I confidently accepted a lucrative and life-changing job offer from a big-time editor—Sir David English (1931-1998)—at a major British newspaper. It was a fabulous opportunity for me to work on London's legendary Fleet Street, join journalism's big league, and to give my sons a spectacular European experience. Both personally and professionally, I was thrilled.

I'm keenly aware that today's working world is light years away from what it was like in the 1980s. Back then, the *Los Angeles Times* used to be known as "The Velvet Coffin" because the employment perks were so generous that few staffers—once hired—ever chose to leave. By accepting the opportunity to relocate to London (and say "Goodbye" to an enviable salary for a journalist, five weeks paid vacation, six sick days and seven holidays each year, free parking, full medical, and dental, and chiropractic insurance coverage, as well as a generous profit-sharing stock program) I became one of a handful of "former" LAT journalists.

***

When honeybees leave their "home," it's always for a very good reason, and is usually triggered when a colony's nest or hive becomes overcrowded. When that happens, the worker bees begin creating larger honeycomb cells for potential new Queens. Once the current Queen lays eggs in those larger structures, the bees that normally forage for nectar slow down their work schedule. At the same time, the Queen stops laying new eggs, and essentially goes on a diet so that it will be easier for her to fly. When she decides the time is right, she will fly out of the hive and be followed by about half of the colony's worker bees. As they leave, they fly together in a large clump (a swarm) that resembles a massive black cloud of loudly buzzing insects.

When the Queen stops—on a tree branch or a lamppost or roof awning—she emits a pheromone that tells the worker bees to cluster around her. They will keep her surrounded for a number of hours while the scout bees scatter in search of a new home. The new residence will rarely be more than one mile away from the nest or hive that they just vacated. As soon as a new location is democratically agreed upon, the workers immediately begin building new honeycomb so that the Queen can resume laying eggs, and pollen and nectar can be stored.

Back at the original hive, new Queens will emerge after spending about two weeks in their cells; the first Queen to emerge will execute the others with her unique reusable stinger. She will then take flight, and mate with drones in order to acquire enough sperm to last for an entire lifespan of daily egg laying.

In areas where there are four seasons, swarming usually happens around the same time when various types of nectar begin to flow. This usually means in the Spring (i.e., from March through May), but swarms can actually form whenever an old colony simply becomes too crowded.

***

So that's how, on a smoggy September morning—it was Labor Day, 1985—my two sons and I (with 27 pieces of luggage) left Los Angeles and moved to London. Before we began the drive to LAX, I made a quick solo visit to each room of our beautiful soon-to-be vacant home. I **walked** over familiar upstairs and downstairs tile and wood and carpeted floors and wished every single room a heartfelt "Thank you," as well as a tentative "Goodbye."

I loved that very pretty house from the very first moment I saw it, back when I was only 25 years old. It wasn't perfect, and it definitely had more than its share of flaws, those "issues" included an itsy-bitsy dining room, a backyard garden that was accessible only by steep concrete steps, and a basement (with a worrisome wooden staircase) that was guaranteed to flood each and every time it rained. But those quirks never diminished the affection I felt for the stately house that I'd proudly thought of as my "forever home."

***

Because traveling is so difficult, I haven't been back to visit that white California colonial since the long-ago day when I closed its front door for the final time. With the help of hindsight and happy memories, I now understand why that house was so important to me; it was because that home was where a much younger, much different, and much healthier me was able to experience so many wonderful moments while I lived there.

That pretty white up-and-down house is where I was strong and young and fit enough to exercise with my boys several times a week. It's where I saw my younger son take his first steps, and where he and his older brother discovered—only twelve miles from the *Los Angeles Times* nine-story building in downtown L.A.—the mysteries and rewards of home-grown flowers and fruits, as well as the rewards of amateur gardening.

Every Fall the boys and I planted 100 bulbs, and every Spring we were surrounded with an explosion of tulips and daffodils and freesias and ranunculus. And those beauties were simply a seasonal addition to our four dozen varieties of vintage rose bushes. Even though I wasn't aware of or obsessed with honeybees back then, what a treat that yard must have been for those local Los Angeles *Apis mellifera*!

Late each sweltering summer (my beloved Colonial home didn't have air conditioning), the boys and I would harvest our backyard bounty—from apricots and plums to peaches and pomegranates and boysenberries. Those heavy buckets of hand-picked fruit became jams and jellies and preserves that would later be carefully carried down the steep basement stairs. They'd then be stored there until added to a schoolyear's worth of peanut butter sandwiches. I can't begin to guess how many hours I was able to stand in our sunny kitchen on my then-strong and healthy legs at either the sink or the stove as our backyard fruit was turned into a homegrown version of Smucker's finest.

***

Today, I'm embarrassed to admit that while my organic fruit trees must have been an ideal destination for pollen and nectar-hungry honeybees, I don't remember ever looking for or seeing them in my garden. At the side of our brick chimney, however, there was a large red Bottlebrush tree that always seemed to have plenty of harmless and happy visiting bees. During all the years I lived in that house, no one was ever stung, and (now that I think of it) in over a decade of living on that property, I don't remember—even once—seeing either a nest or a hive. Obviously, my fruit-bearing trees (as well as my flower-filled front yard) were blessed with very well-behaved visiting (i.e., foraging and pollinating) honeybees.

For over 50 years, I've enjoyed an amazing friendship with the artist and author Donna Brown Agins. She recently reminded me of a long ago Summer afternoon when we were sitting together in the backyard patio, and discussing her upcoming trip to Paris. While I had completely forgotten the details of our conversation, she clearly remembers that I had placed my chair in front of a cluster of rose bushes that were in full bloom. As we talked, an industrious group of honeybees continually circled around the nearby flowers that must have been overflowing with nectar. Donna remembers that there were always lots of buzzing honeybees hovering near my flower garden, but they paid no attention to us whatsoever. I wonder if they presciently knew that someday in the far-distant future I would be one of their biggest fans…

***

The same way that the hive is the place where honeybees learn their different skills, that lovely house was the home base from which I learned how to hang wallpaper, resuscitate tarnished brass or silver, as well as paint and refinish wooden furniture. Like a doting overprotective guardian, I worried about our beautiful home's long list of needs, and I was determined to learn how to do whatever it took to bring out and showcase its aging and authentic charms.

Unfortunately, during the years when the domestic goddess wannabe side of me was figuring out how to unstick the garbage disposal with a broom handle or use geometry-class skills to measure and sew bedspreads, curtains and seat covers, my marriage crumbled and fell apart. The house that had once been my source of contentment and pride, also became my refuge for the comfort and peace my shattered heart needed in order to heal.

After our divorce, I found myself—in my late 20s with two adorable little boys who needed me—in a state of pure terror about what the future held for us. It's funny how those emotionally anxious (but young and healthy and physically fit) times now seem as if they were my life's "good old days." Just as the Queen Bee has no authority figure to turn to, I had no parents or siblings to rely on either. So, instead, I took comfort from the sturdy walls of that pretty white up-and-down house to give me a sense of stability and strength. My much-loved home never once disappointed me.

That beautiful two-story structure absorbed my single-mother sorrow, and it calmed my shaken sense of security. As I shuffle through my decades-old motherhood memories, I recall the warmth I felt whenever my sons and I were in the car together, and we'd turn onto our street. Whether we were returning from an out-of-town trip, or just driving back from the stables or the ice rink, I always found myself sighing with relief and smiling as our cherished home came into view. I know how much the honeybees care for (and about) their homes, and I wonder if they also feel comfort and joy when their hives come into view.

***

Years later, while I lived in London, a local real estate company leased out our home, but by the time I'd returned to the States and settled in Florida, there was a long list of expensive structural repairs that could no longer be postponed. By then, I was fighting MS, unemployed (not to mention unemployable), living off my miniscule savings, and there was no way I could afford to fix our beloved home's construction problems. The heart-wrenching grim truth was that my pretty white up-and-down house would have to be sold. On one of the saddest days of my life, I sat in my wheelchair in front of a local Florida notary public, and repeatedly (and tearfully) signed the fat stack of papers that meant someone else—a fortunate stranger—would soon own my beautiful California home.

Today, I live in a small palm tree-shaded bungalow in South Florida. There is no vista of a mountain range, no basement, no beautiful marble fireplace, no fruit trees, and no rose garden. Instead, there are wide, wheelchair-friendly doorways, plus hand grips and ramps rather than inside and outdoor stairways. Now, the little boys I raised in that pretty white up-and-down house are grown men who have beautiful homes and lovely families of their own. Today, I'm painfully aware that I foolishly took my youthful health and my astonishing good fortune for granted.

Each time I glance at the framed and well—traveled photo of that once laughter and music—filled house, I can't help but smile. I always find it comforting to know that even though I can't physically go back to that time or to that place, for a few short years the sweetest home imaginable was once well and truly mine.

WHAT THE HONEYBEES TAUGHT ME

- For both humans and honeybees, life is always full of changes. The lyricist Helen Deutsch (1906-1992) captured that sentiment perfectly when she wrote *"Nothing is forever, always is a lie."* In other words, life is continually on the move.
- I've had valuables stolen from my homes in Los Angeles, London, and West Palm Beach, and it's helped me relate to how *Apis mellifera* must feel when we routinely raid their honey supplies. We may lose valuable items during our lifetime, but—thank goodness—no one can steal our cherished memories.
- It's always a good idea to surround yourself—in your garden or in your home—with as many flowers and plants and trees as possible.
- *Apis mellifera's* magic should remind us that not all the powerful forces at work in your garden—or in your life—are obvious or visible.
- As Virgil (70 BC-19 BC) observed, *Tempus fugit* (in other words, time really does fly).

- Even if you're oblivious (as I was) regarding all the amazing things that honeybees do to enhance your life, they are still always (literally, always) hard at work on your behalf.

Chapter 4
Work, Work, Work, Work, Work

No matter how hard you work, someone else is working harder.

Elon Musk

There is a good reason why the phrase "Busy as a bee" has become part of our lexicon. It would be hard to find any other creature on Earth that works so enthusiastically and industriously for its entire lifespan. Because honeybees are so small, it's easy to forget just how driven they are and how much they accomplish in such a short time.

During a worker bee's short lifespan, her wings will work at the rate of 200 beats per second, and she will be able to fly close to 15 miles per hour. The mature bees who fly outside the hive and forage for nectar are each able to produce about 1/12th of a teaspoon of honey during their entire 45-day lifespan. Worker bees usually die because their fragile translucent wings literally get worn out after only a few weeks spent working so hard and flying so far.

***

When I look around these days, I can't help but notice that many of the people I come in contact with—unlike the honeybees—seem to have what I would call a bifurcated lifestyle. Most of my friends tend to have one side of life that includes their professional accomplishments, and then a different side that is merely an avocation or a hobby. For example, Paul is a brilliant attorney, but when he's not arguing cases he can be found tending to his impressive orchid collection. Another friend of mine has had a great career as a real estate agent, but whenever she has free time she loves to work creating beautiful collages. And my friend, Angela, is a gifted teacher by day, but when she's not helping her students, she loves to create beautiful clothes on her sewing machine.

When I first encountered the concept of having two major outlets—one professional and one personal—I was somewhat taken aback because it was so different from the way I was raised. When I was in high school, my parents' lifestyle was dramatically different from what my peers experienced, and it added to my uncomfortable feeling of being a teenager who was undeniably "different" than her classmates.

Part of the reason that my adolescence was unusual is that my parents were on their honeymoon when *The Great Depression* began in October 1929. The subsequent Stock Market crash had a profoundly negative effect on millions of individuals, and my parents were among those who suffered unfortunate life-long repercussions from that economic nightmare.

One of the effects of losing their—and their families'—financial stability at such a young age was that for the rest of their lives my parents were consistently frugal, fiercely independent, and resourceful. For them, it was emotionally essential to always be both resilient and self-sufficient.

I'm proud to say that my father was a man of his pre-WWII generation. He took quiet pride in the fact that he could rely on his own skills to fix whatever might go wrong at home—wherever we happened to live. During my childhood, I never once saw a repairman enter our home. On weekends, Daddy could (and happily did) fix anything and everything—whether it was a broken toaster or a leaky roof. From Monday through Friday, his office wardrobe consisted of *Mad Men*-era dark suits, conservative ties, and Oxblood lace-up Oxfords. But on Saturday and Sunday, he loved to wear chinos and "too old" dress shirts that would routinely absorb garden stains, grease spills, or paint splatters.

My mother, also from the same generation, was a tiny Kentucky-born woman who scorned the idea of leisure time. She loved being productive, and took great pride in her various domestic skills, which ranged from making pies to baking fresh loaves of bread, to canning her home-grown vegetables, as well as embroidering pillowcases or making her own quilts.

Additionally–without complaint—she cooked three separate meals every day of her married life. No matter where we lived, my father always drove home from work to have a hot lunch with her each day because (in their opinion) it would have been "a waste of money" to pay for a mediocre meal when they could share a tastier one at home together.

In high school, my friends loved to go shopping with their mothers because it meant being able to return home with the latest Lanz nightgown or maybe a new pair of Pappagallos. But I never had that sort of retail bonding experience with my mother—because she was easily 20 years older than my friends' moms—and would be appalled at both the prices and the workmanship of the things I so desperately wanted to own. Dismissively, she would say, *"Oh, for heaven's sake. I could make this twice as nice for half the cost."* As a result, I would return home embarrassed and emptyhanded, but determined to find a way to somehow—independently—get whatever it was that I wanted to purchase.

Part of their parenting philosophy was the belief that they needed to teach me as many necessary "life skills" as possible so that I (like them) would be able to enjoy a self-reliant adulthood. Mama saw to it that I—an obedient but only mildly appreciative apprentice—learned how to knit my own sweaters, sew my own clothes, cook a tasty meal, and do whatever else she envisioned that married life might one day ask of me. Back then, we didn't have Google to answer questions that began with "How do I. . . ," so our adolescent years were spent accruing abilities, practical skills, and ways to better navigate through adulthood.

As a result, I became a woman who was able to convince myself that I could stand on my own two feet, and adequately accomplish whatever needed to be done by myself. I placed a very high emotional premium on both my so-called independence and self-defined productive abilities.

***

Part of my gradual immersion into the honeybee world, was that I had to recalibrate the reverence that I'd always had for my imagined independence. Watching the continual activity within a beehive showed me that female worker bees seemed to have been born with an incredible changing and evolving set of skills. Honeybees live in what is essentially an "Eusocial unit," which means that each individual honeybee behaves as an individual that is an essential part of a larger organic whole. The inhabitants of a beehive seem to be born with the knowledge that no one can survive by themselves for very long. Honeybee colonies rely on each and every one of its thousands of workers just as crucially as it needs its extremely essential Queen Bee.

The honeybee hive is multi-generational; it includes adult, offspring, as well as gestating eggs, and one of the things that make the eusocial unit so unique is that all of the female worker bees take part in a continually rotating division of labor. For an allotted period of time, each honeybee has a clearly-defined role. The community's macro division includes the Queen, thousands of worker bees, and a handful of drones. On the other hand, the micro division includes builders, undertakers, scouts, guards, nursery workers, honey processors, hive, and honeycomb cleaners, as well as—a honeybee's final

58

job—hunting for and retrieving both nectar and pollen.

Even more amazing than the sheer variety of their jobs is the fact that worker bees appear to have some sort of internal clock that controls the evolution and scheduling of how they contribute to the smooth functioning of the hive. Here is a glimpse of their ever-evolving changing careers:

All honeybees begin as an egg that the queen has laid at the bottom of a honeycomb structure made of hexagonal cells. Essentially, after three days, the egg hatches and turns into a larva, where it is then fed Royal Jelly from nurse bees. After six more days of gestation, it enters an "inactive pupa" stage, which lasts for the next twelve days.

On the 21st day, the fully-formed worker will exit the honeycomb cell, and begin a 45-day long lifetime of astounding productivity. She and her sisters will do absolutely everything that needs to be done in and for the hive or nest—with the exclusion of becoming impregnated and laying eggs. Here's a look at their continually changing chronological assignments:

- Days 1 and 2: **Janitorial work**. After the newborns consume lots of honey and pollen, the hungry worker bees leave their cells for the first time. Then, during the first two days of life, the worker bees will carefully clean the honeycomb cells they've just left. This must be accomplished before the Queen visits and prepares to lay a new series of additional replacement eggs. Since the Queen is a perfectionist, each hexagonal area must be completely antiseptic.

- Days 3 through 12: **Young nurse**. At this age, a young worker bee's life is spent feeding the developing larvae. These youthful worker bees create a form of nourishment known as Royal Jelly, which is secreted from their internal glands. The nurse bees work tirelessly—over 1,000 times a day—to ensure that the larvae will be healthy.

The human equivalent (at least based on my age as a septuagenarian) would be around eight years old, which for most girls is essentially "playing with dolls" time. As much as I like to fantasize that my life mirrors a bee's, when I was a little girl (much to my mother's dismay) I had very little interest in dolls. In fact, the only doll I ever loved was over three feet tall, and I used her to create and construct my idea of a "perfect" wardrobe of clothes cobbled together from my mother's fabric remnants.

- Days 3 through 16: **Mortuary bees**. These worker bees are tasked with the job of removing dead larvae and deceased bees from the hive. Mortuary bees frequently carry these corpses as far away from the hive as possible in order to prevent disease, and they will sometimes fly 20 feet away from the hive with a bee corpse before dropping it to the ground. If the dead bee is too big or heavy the mortuary bees will slowly drag the corpse out of the hive and then push it to the ground below, which becomes a convenient—but undesirable—local honeybee cemetery. When necessary, mortuary bees deal with dead hive invaders by covering their corpses with propolis.

- Days 4 through 12: **Drone feeder**. Each colony raises a few hundred to a few thousand drones in case a new virgin Queen will need to be inseminated. The drones are never popular because (unlike the worker bees) they only have one job, and contribute nothing else to the overall wellbeing of the hive. Usually, their more rectangular-shaped bodies sets them apart from the thousands of females in the hive.
- Days 6 through 12: **Experienced nurse**. Some of the nurse bees care for the larvae that have been set aside to potentially become either Queen Bees—who only receive Royal Jelly for their entire lives—or a few hundred drones or several hundred worker bees who (after their first three days of life) receive a mixture of pollen and other nutrients. The "nurses" who care for the Queen Bee literally do everything for her – including even the removal of her excrement.

Worker bees of this age will begin their jobs of caring for, feeding, and grooming the Queen Bee. This allows them to be exposed to (and then spread) the Queen's mandibular pheromone (QMP) throughout the hive. When the workers deliver her unique fragrance, it lets the rest of the hive's 60,000 honeybees know the physical status of their Queen.

Again, my life trajectory definitely did not mesh with what a worker bee would be doing at this stage. A twelve-day-old bee would be considered an experienced nurse, and many of my classmates from the Catholic girls' high school that I attended did go on to become registered nurses. I, however, was the only girl in our class who had no interest whatsoever in becoming a volunteer hospital candy striper. In my twenties and thirties, however, I cared passionately about the body and physical wellbeing , until my own health was in freefall.

- Days 7 through 22: **Pollen packers**. After foraging, the older bees bring nectar, pollen and propolis back to the hive and each product gets processed into specific uses. An enzyme gets added to the freshly-delivered nectar, and the bees inside the hive fan the holding cells to evaporate enough water to turn the nectar into honey. The pollen that they bring to the nest or hive can be used to feed the brood, but it can also be stored for the colony's future food needs. The bees with this task pack down the pollen into honeycomb cells, and then mix it with a small amount of honey so that it never spoils. (Without a small amount of anti-bacterial honey, stored pollen can become rancid.)

  In my own life, this stage would be similar to the time when I was collecting cookbooks; I once had over one hundred volumes. I loved inviting people to our home for brunches or dinner parties, and making garden-fresh jams and jellies. Unlike the honeybees, we never had to worry about "running out of" food (i.e. nectar, pollen, or honey), but I still took the concept of planning "event meals" far more seriously than I needed to.

- Days 12 through 18: **Airconditioning bees**. Climate control honeybees have an astonishing ability to keep the environment in the hive (or nest) at a consistent temperature of around 93 degrees. The workers control the warmth of the hive by using their four wings to control airflow into, out of, as well as within the beehive.

- Days 12 through 18: **Water carrier**. Foraging worker bees find water on damp rocks, muddy puddles, branches, and even as dew that rests on plants and leaves. They swallow the water and store it in their (throat) crops before they fly home to transfer water into the mouths of thirsty workers waiting inside the hive. This direct exchange of water from one honeybee to another is called *tropahallaxios*.

While honeybees have no way to store water inside their hive, they are able to spread moisture on top of sealed brood or even on the backs of other parched A/C bees that may be in danger of getting overheated. Tiny droplets of water are used to make sure that the Queen (as well as the rest of the hive inhabitants) will be well-hydrated. During fifth, sixth, and seventh grade.

I attended Immaculate Conception elementary school in Yuma, Arizona. Before that, we had lived in California and Oregon, where we had never been forced to think about the importance of water. But living in the middle of a triple-digit hot and arid desert had a life-long impact on my relationship with H_2O. Those three years taught me something that honeybees have known since the beginning of time, which is that water—or the lack thereof— can be the difference between life and death.

- Days 12 through 18: **Wax makers**. This group of bees make wax and build honeycombs. The beeswax—which is produced by four specific abdominal glands—allows these worker bees to repair old damaged cells, and create additional hexagons to house new eggs. The honeycomb is also used to store both nectar and pollen that has been brought to the hive by the more mature (i.e., older) workers. Creating beeswax and building honeycomb are essential duties for the bees' survival.

- Days 13 through 35: **Wax workers**. Bees that seal the filled honeycombs serve a valuable purpose because those reservoirs of honey are what keep the colony's population nourished when the weather is cold and/or when there is little or no nectar to be found. The residue that is used to seal the honeycomb is referred to as "Cap," and many *Apis mellifera* fans consider it to be a valuable part of the health-giving world of bee products.

  The human equivalent would be planning financially for the future by maintaining a healthy savings account. Once upon a time (believe it or not), I had a robust 401k plan, a decent stock portfolio, and a good-sized savings account, but they all disappeared when my health imploded, my earning ability evaporated, and my medical expenses exploded. Sadly, when it comes to chronic illnesses there are no budgetary bargains. The good news is, I'm slowly inching my way back into financial respectability…

- Days 18 through 21: **Guard bees**. Posted at the hive entrance, these defensive honeybees are tasked with keeping other insects or predators out of the hive. The number of a colony's protective guard bees depends on weather conditions, the hive's population, the amount of air traffic present, and how aggressive the attackers are.

- Days 18 through 21: **Mite fighters**. When small hive beetles or Varroa mites do manage to enter and infect the honeybee community, a small number of SWAT-team worker bees will engage in a form of "group confinement behavior." This method of surrounding, isolating, and ultimately destroying a hive's enemy is an effective way to protect the other bees as well as their home.

Unlike the honeybees, I don't think I've ever managed to proactively "destroy" anything. But during my first years of being a single mother, I do remember feeling hyper-vigilant about a wide variety of real and potential catastrophic possibilities. I'm happy to say that none of those imagined frightening scenarios ever came to pass, but a part of me definitely regrets wasting so much precious energy on *"what if"* make-belief horrors.

- Days 18 through 45: **Propolis gatherers**. At this age, worker bees can gather resin from tree bark and certain plants; they then add enzymes that turns the resin into an antibacterial/antifungal form of beehive "concrete" called propolis. This unique bee product substance can be used by the honeybees to mummify invaders, as well as to seal and repair any unwanted openings in the hive's walls.

By the time I had reached this "stage" in my life, MS was totally in charge of my life. Unlike the foraging bees, who can fly as far as six miles away from their hive if necessary, at that point (in my 40s)

I was unable to go anywhere without the help of kind souls who were willing to assist me.

- Days 22 through 45: **Hunters and Scouts**. Essential foragers (who search for nectar, pollen, and propolis) as well as, the scouts (that hunt for a swarm's new home) can travel several miles away from the hive or nest in order to complete their assigned task.

In summary, the first two days of a worker bee's life revolves around janitorial duty. The next two or three days will be spent caring for brood larvae, the next five days involve royal caretaking, and the week after that will be spent building or distributing bee-essential necessities. The next several days of their short lifespan will be spent guarding the hive, taking care of the inner air temperature, and removing the bodies of deceased sisters from the hive. From the third week of life until its end (which usually happens around the 40th day) is spent primarily outside of the hive searching for nectar, pollen, resin, water, or a suitable new nest.

WHAT THE HONEYBEES TAUGHT ME

- Honeybees have always known how to make the most of what little time they have on this earth. As Charles Darwin (1809-1882) wrote *"A man who dares to waste one hour of time has not discovered the value of life."* Essentially, life is too short for them (or you) to waste time. It's much more gratifying to be productive.
- *Apis mellifera* know that it's always okay to ask others for help when you need it. And others—insects

66

and humans alike—often relish the opportunity to be (and feel) needed.

- Because we never know what surprises fate might have in store for us, the more skills and abilities you can accrue in your lifetime, the better.

- If you're lucky, one day you might be able to see hundreds of bees tumble out of their hive entrance, almost like schoolchildren who have been dismissed from the classroom. These are younger bees who are—together—leaving the hive for the very first time, and testing out their unproven wings. Their days of working inside the hive are over, and they can now join the all-important foragers who bring the hive's food supply and much-needed water back to their hardworking sisters.

- The continual and cooperative activity of a beehive is a perfect illustration of John Donne's (1572-1631) observation that *"No man* [or honeybee] *is an island entire of itself* [or herself]."

- The amazing and accomplished Helen Keller (1880-1968), who was both blind and deaf, wasn't talking about honeybees but was right when she said, *"Alone we can do so little—together we can do so much."*

Chapter 5
Beeswax

*Great things are done by a series of small things
brought together.*

Vincent Van Gogh (1853-1890)

In the 1980s, which was when Baby Boomers (like me) were in our heyday, the adjective of choice was BIG. Shoulder pads, hairstyles, the economy, Tom Hanks' hit movie—you name it—the overwhelming message seemed to be that bigger was definitely better. The phrase "Go big or go home" had become the accepted aphorism of that long-ago time.

No one has ever called me a "shrinking violet," but I simply never had the necessary self-confidence to wholeheartedly embrace anything that seemed larger-than-life. I had plenty of peers who were very comfortable being a big fish in a small pond, but I much preferred to be a small fish in a big pond.

The more I thought about it, the more I realized that my inner sense of comfort regarding small things probably had a lot to do with my fondness for the different types of detailed needlework that I'd learned back in elementary school. From crocheting to knitting to sewing my own clothes, I grew to treasure the fact that tiny stitches—when combined—could create an endless number of items that were attractive, functional, and (occasionally) essential. And after I learned how to needlepoint—thanks to the patient guidance of my dear friend Toni Sherman—small color-filled stitches became an everyday part of my life.

When I read Sutton Foster's memoir *Hooked: How Crafting Saved My Life*, I immediately identified with the feelings she experienced whenever she held a needle in her words, "*In my family, we didn't talk about our emotions... I wanted something that I could pour my love into [and] each item I made could be an act of love... Every stitch got me that much closer to a revelation. I was...an extrovert in my personal life... I needed this quiet contemplation in order to perform well.*"

Over the years, I've needlepointed belts, chair covers, footstools, pillows, purses, rugs, wall hangings, as well as a variety of Christmas stockings and tree ornaments for those I love. I've never taken the time to compute how many stitches I've made over the last half-century, but I'm willing to wager that the number would run in the multimillions.

Twenty-five years ago, motivated by the scary thought that I might lose the use of both my hands, I began to catalog my canvas and yarn creations. Today, I have a 8x9 inch photo album that is three inches thick with over 200 snapshots of completed small-stitch projects that commemorates my 50-year needlepoint addiction.

***

When I began to study the different fascinating aspects of the *Apis mellifera* world, my attention didn't immediately go to honey or to the social dynamics of hive inhabitants. Instead, it went to beeswax, primarily because its all-natural origin is one of the tiniest components of the honeybees' home base. Many people feel that honey (or pollen or propolis or royal jelly) is the most important bee product there is, but without the wax that makes the honeycomb, nothing in the bee world would be possible.

***

When I think of those little worker bees (who are about the size of the fingernail of your ring finger) I flash back to my years—fifth, sixth, and seventh grade—when my mother was worried that her horse-crazy daughter was becoming too much of a tomboy. Instead of sending me to Cotillion classes, she arranged for me to spend six hours each week with three older (and very gifted) needlewomen.

I could walk to their yarn shop (which was actually in the converted living room of their home) after school. Wearing my blue and white Immaculate Conception elementary school uniform, I would try to balance my school books and my black violin case as I rang their doorbell every Tuesday and Thursday afternoon. Once inside their crowded shop, I'd settle in for an hour-long one-on-one class. If my memory is correct, Tuesday afternoons were for knitting lessons with Miss Abigail and Thursdays were for learning how to crochet with Miss Edith. My grandmotherly instructors were patient, encouraging, and kind, and I loved the fact that they always made me feel as if my afternoon arrival was the favorite part of their day. The knitted socks that I made for my father and the crocheted doilies I made for my mother disappeared decades ago, but the County Fair ribbons that I won are still glued into my now-disintegrating adolescent scrapbook.

Saturday mornings were reserved for sewing lessons at the local Singer Sewing machine shop. Miss Jeanette who—in a few short months—taught pre-teen girls the subtle but important distinction between "getting dressed" and simply "putting on clothes." She made sure that we knew the different types of fabrics (from Brocade to Chiffon to Dotted Swiss to Taffeta). I truly cherished my scheduled classes with those three talented women, each of whom happily accepted the challenge of teaching (often clueless and clumsy) young girls what they felt were essential life skills.

From the plastic containers where I now keep all my yarns organized by color and type, to the different groups of needles, as well as the various types and sizes of needlepoint canvas, everything about the structure and creation of beeswax and honeycomb feels familiar and cozy.

***

Most people (including me) wouldn't know that, after the Romans captured Corsica in the second century BC, they had very little interest in commandeering the island's valuable honey reserves.

71

Instead, they demanded a "tribute" of 200,000 pounds of beeswax every year. Why? Because back then beeswax was used for everything from candles and lamp oil to medications, and it was even an essential component of the ancient era's version of an erasable whiteboard.

Today, when most of us think of beeswax, what usually comes to mind first are the pricey and natural non-drip, clean-burning aromatic honeycomb candles. One of the reasons that candles from beeswax are so special is that they last (i.e., burn) much longer than common candles, which are usually derived from petroleum (i.e., paraffin). They also provide stronger light because they burn brighter, are cleaner, and are also smokeless. Part of the reason for their superiority is that beeswax has a higher melting point than any other candle-making ingredient. So, while these candles may seem more costly, in fact, they are a far more sensible choice.

Historically, beeswax has been remarkable versatile and—throughout history—it has been used for a wide variety of other purposes. Religious orders used beeswax exclusively for worship service candles, but as beekeeping began to be a more secular activity its popularity grew far beyond cloistered monastery walls.

One of the more unusual applications for beeswax was—musically—to hold together the reeds used in wind instruments; it's also been used as the drumroll of a tambourine or as a fine resin for wooden string instruments. Beeswax has also played a role in what is known as Cutlers resin, which can also include pine pitch (as well as bits of sawdust), and was used to attach blades onto knife handles. For centuries, carpenters and woodworkers have used beeswax to eliminate squeaks, smooth out cabinet drawers, keep screws in place, and highlight the luster of various grains of wood.

On a more macabre note, I was recently told that centuries ago melted beeswax was often used to sculpt face masks of the deceased. Rumor has it that Madame Tussaud's legendary career began when (in 1793) she used beeswax to capture the images of the guillotined Marie Antoinette and Louis the XVI.

While honeycomb and beeswax candles do have a costly and refined elegance, their origins are far less romantic. Beeswax actually begins as tiny liquid pellets that are secreted from four pairs of wax glands located on the underside of the very young— during the first two weeks of their lives—worker bee's abdomen. Worker bees start to secrete wax about 12 days after they emerge from their honeycomb cell. After only six days those glands degenerate, and that particular worker bee will have "aged out," and no longer be able to produce usable wax.

Those miniscule secretions have been compared to a form of *Apis mellifera* "dandruff." In a 12-hour block of time, a young worker bee can deposit about eight bits of wax. Although they begin as a liquid, once the scales are exposed to air, they begin to harden. A normal hive (or nest) needs about 1,000 waxy bits to make a single gram of beeswax;

once the wax hardens, the process of building honeycomb begins in earnest.

Like almost everything else involved in the honeybee world, in spite of our modern scientific abilities, beeswax—like royal jelly, propolis, and even honey—simply cannot be synthetically reproduced in a laboratory. Beeswax has over 300 different components that range from aromatic esters, hydrocarbons, minerals, and a variety of other ingredients. And while 75% of beeswax is comprised of a variety of alcohols, including palmitic and malefic, it also contains oleic acids. Beeswax dissolves easily in gas, turpentine, or any other strong acidic substance. Surprisingly, there is four times more Vitamin A in beeswax than is found in carrots, which might be one reason why beeswax has become an essential ingredient for a variety of both medical and cosmetic products.

In ancient times, beeswax was frequently used for its wound-healing abilities, and the original physicians Avicenna (980 CE-1037 CE) and Hippocrates (460 BC-375 BC) both believed that beeswax was a natural panacea that could help everyone from breastfeeding new mothers to asthmatics, ulcer sufferers, and even patients with chronic digestive problems. Through the years, beeswax has also been useful for a variety of non-medicinal purposes. For example, cheesemakers used beeswax for centuries as a coating to deter mold or spoilage, and in today's world it can also be found in everything from lip balms to body lotions.

Archaeologists have discovered that Egyptians made beeswax candles as far back as the sixth century.

In a full year, a single hive can generate seven kilograms (or 16 pounds) of wax, which is amazing when you think of how miniscule each small flake is, and that it takes about 400,000 of them—almost half a million—just to make one pound of beeswax.

Because of its ability to effectively tolerate heat, beeswax is a substance that can be stored for hundreds of years without losing its beneficial properties. Its has a melting point of 148°F, and doesn't become stiff or brittle until the temperature drops to about 60 degrees. This allows honeycomb to tolerate a wide range of different climates.

In today's beauty business and medical world, beeswax is primarily used in creams, masks, ointments, and patches. Hippocrates (460 BC-370 BC) suggested using beeswax to help anyone who suffered from throat issues, and some modern acupuncturists place melted beeswax on specific meridian points to help stimulate the circulatory system. This may be one reason why beeswax is rumored to improve athletic or muscular performance.

Also, some apitherapy practitioners apply hot beeswax to relieve osteochondrosis as well as arthritis pain, and several use wax packs (which include honey and pollen) to treat patients with painful polyarthritis. Many beekeepers also swear that chewing honeycomb is also helpful for overcoming fatigue; swallowing what remains of the once honey-filled beeswax is considered to be an easy way to first soothe the gums, and then help the digestive system.

***

Essentially, beeswax is like the brick and mortar of a beehive (or a bee nest). It takes about eight pounds of nectar for the young worker bees to make one pound of beeswax. Although the wax itself starts out soft and pliable, the hexagonal structure of honeycomb is actually exceptionally strong, and it makes the perfect six-sided storage space for honey, larvae, and pollen. When it comes to my personal passion for tiny or small spaces that need to be filled—i.e., needlepoint—the varieties of sizes can range from 22 stitches per inch (*petit point*) to much larger stitches. Sometimes the canvas can be as large as five stitches per inch, which just so happens to be the exact same dimension as beeswax honeycomb cells.

As mentioned earlier, the wax is secreted from glands under the young worker bee's abdomen, and the tiny clear damp pieces that fall off resemble miniature old-fashioned Ivory Soap flakes. Those miniscule waxy bits then get heated—in the hive or in the nest—to almost 90 degrees as part of the honeycomb-making process.

Worker honeybees have three sets of two legs—one set is at the rear of the body, one is in the middle, and one (almost like arms) is at the front of its body. She uses the stiff hairs on her hind legs to remove any pollen or wax residue from her abdomen, and then the tiny flakes get transferred from one set of legs to the next until they reach the worker bee's mouth. That's where the flakes get chewed, change color from transparent to a soft white color, and then—once it is transferred—the wax is ready to begin its future as part of the honeycomb shape. The softened chewed wax is measured and molded by the worker bee's mouth into the "correct" thickness, and then it is molded into the hexagonal shape as part of a joint construction activity.

Only the bodies of very young *Apis mellifera*—who never leave the hive for the first two weeks of their lives—are able to create wax deposits. As the days pass, their as-yet-unused wings gradually get stronger, and they are finally able to fly. When that happens, their wax-making glands simultaneously stop processing their translucent material, and become inactive.

* * *

Back when I was 22 years old, part of the reason that I was drawn to needlepoint was that it seemed to be a totally decorative (rather than practical) activity. Up to that point, so much of my life had been focused on achievement, productivity, and being useful, that I was intrigued by the idea of a creative pastime that allowed me to think solely in terms of visual appeal.

During the 1970s, there were lots of small needlepoint shops in the Los Angeles area that were overflowing with colorful yarns. The textured cotton, silk, and wool offerings made entering a small retail store feel like walking inside a magical and colorful flower garden. When the high cost of hand-painted canvases became prohibitive, I decided to learn how to create and customize my own needlepoint projects by "borrowing" ideas from counted cross-stitch patterns. All I had to do was pay (very) close attention to the number of squares on each design element, and then "paint" the selected scenery or chosen words that I wanted to replicate by using my old treasured friends: a shiny needle and carefully chosen colorful yarn.

For decades, I've been mildly obsessive about trying to keep all my yarns organized by color, so that whether I needed several strands of a pale pink or lots of a deep burgundy or a small amount of metallic midnight blue yarn, my choices were always easy to find. For each needlepoint project, I would rely on a plastic "butterfly-shaped" palette-size yarn holder with holes that let me keep all my selected colors easily at hand. I learned to enjoy the lengthy "prep work" of organizing my supplies long before I ever made the first stitch on a new project.

For me, there has always been something about working with canvas and colorful yarn—plus the potential creation of something truly beautiful—that I found automatically calming and rewarding. For decades, needlepoint has been a tangible and visible form of meditation that can instantaneously lower my blood pressure and allow me to (temporarily) feel accomplished and serene, even when every other aspect of my life seems chaotic and out of control.

***

The amount of wax that the bees produce is actually determined by how much nectar the older foraging bees bring back home. If the returning worker bees have too much nectar stored in their stomachs, some sort of inexplicable signal goes out to the youngsters in the hive, and their wax-making glands go into overdrive. It's almost as if the hive becomes a changeable high-tech assembly line that continually operates via an atmospheric feedback that allows the "honey-making factory" to speed up, slow down, and run smoothly without any supply-side disruptions.

When the bees build their honeycomb, they do it—just as with practically everything in the hives—as a group effort. Like a living form of insect macrame, strings of young workers form an interconnected and acrobatic "chain" of active *Apis mellifera*. Clustered together as a group, they create the necessary heat to mold and construct the hexagonal honeycomb pods, which are called "cells." Each one is built to exacting measurements, and since the hive's needs change periodically, the size and capacity of the wax structure can adapt as needed.

The industrious worker bees first build honeycomb in perfectly vertical lines, and (like everything else in the hive) this construction project takes place in the dark. Since they can't see whether or not the connection is straight, each honeybee locks her legs with another hive inhabitant in order to create a perfect plumbline. Then, a single worker bee arrives at the spot where the honeycomb will begin. And, after that, a straight line of worker bee bodies (with their legs connected to one another) help direct their helpful sisters to create a straight line—from the top of the frame all the way to the bottom—of beeswax honeycomb.

Five of those small carefully-crafted beeswax hexagons will fit into a one-inch space, and a single pound of beeswax will contain an impressive 35,000 of those individual cells. And while the wax used to build the connected cells may have started out as a moist "flake," by the time the honeycomb is formed and filled, it is strong enough to easily hold about 15 pounds of honey.

The worker bees that construct the honeycomb cells seem to also instinctively know another essential detail: each cell is slightly tilted upward as a way to prevent stored honey from spilling out. Somehow, *Apis mellifera* know that pointing the honeycomb cells upwards at a 13 degree angle will do the job perfectly. I have no idea how they calibrate the correct angle of every single cell, but I do know that the six-sided shape is stronger than any other geometric option (like triangles, rectangles or squares). Those very precise perfectly-constructed wax cells are also able to provide honeybees with the largest and strongest possible storage area.

Inside the modern wooden hives that are so popular today, many beekeepers use a lightweight sheet of wax-covered plastic to create a hexagonal foundation for the creation of honeycomb. These are often referred to as "starters" because they help worker bees construct the essential architecture of the honeycomb. This plastic wax foundation resembles a single sheet of construction paper, and the worker bees create honeycomb by building on top of its subtle hexagonal outlines. The resulting cells can then be used as a place for the Queen to lay her eggs, a place for the baby bees to gestate, or as a storage unit for honey. If a bee nest or a hive is left to its own devices, a honeycomb layer or frame will usually have larvae clustered in the center; cells full of honey (or pollen) will either surround it or be placed around the outer edges.

More sophisticated beekeeping often involves the use of a Queen Excluder, which prevents the Queen (who is larger than her worker bee daughters) from entering and laying eggs on specific honeycomb frames. By keeping the honey and the larvae receptacles separate, beekeepers can more easily "harvest" their sweet crop without damaging the next gestating generation of bees. Once the honeycomb is built and filled with honey, a beekeeper can then remove the frame—without harming brood—by using a tool known as a "hot knife" that melts the propolis seal that keeps it shut.

*** *** ***

As I've mentioned before every single case of MS is different. For me, the first two frightening symptoms came when the soles of both my feet began to feel strange. I could still walk, but the bottoms of my feet felt "round." (It almost seemed as if I were walking with Idaho potatoes below my ankles, instead of on the soles of my own two feet.) That strange sensation lasted for about a month. Then, my entire right foot refused to function as it should have; the medical term for what I experienced is called "drop foot."

Within a matter of months I developed a slight limp, and soon afterwards my left leg began to sporadically grow weaker and weaker. After a concerted effort to clean up my diet, flood my system with supplements, and receive frequent chiropractic adjustments, I entered a blissful state of symptom-free remission.

I was still in that giddy state of *"Wow, I just dodged a big bullet, which must mean I'm the luckiest girl in the world,"* when I received the golden-ticket invitation to join the staff of a big-time London newspaper. I—being a Stubborn Optimist—jumped at the opportunity, and moved 6,000 miles away from my support system and every single aspect of my life that was comforting, familiar, and safe.

Six weeks after moving to the U.K., my boys and I were returning to our flat in Notting Hill, and walking together along Kensington High Street on a beautiful Saturday afternoon. Without warning, both my legs began to tingle and feel strange, and soon afterwards, the dreaded limp resurfaced. For the next three years, I was able to work and travel and live a relatively normal life because I acted as if I were dealing with a "muscle spasm" or a "pinched nerve" or any other random explanation that would allow me to convince myself (and others) that I didn't really have MS.

By 1989, I was no longer able to fool myself—or anyone else—about my failing health. There was no way I could possibly ignore the fact that there was definitely something seriously and progressively wrong with my body. Again, every case of MS is unique, but (for me) the slow downward trajectory included (four years after that brisk but heartbreaking lunchtime diagnosis) the feeling that each of my legs weighed about 500 pounds. Every step involved concentration and conscious (often exhausting and painful) effort.

***

It's no secret that I love everything about London. But at that time, I did whatever I could—at friends' homes, movie theaters, restaurants, the underground (aka "The Tube"), even doctors' offices—to avoid the inevitable annoying presence of up-and-down stairs. It seemed as if anywhere and everywhere I went I would be confronted with some sort of staircase configuration that would require lifting one deeply resistant leg after the other in order to reach my desired destination. As a result, I left my flat less and less often, which meant that I became more alone and isolated than I'd ever been in my entire life.

Day after day, I was living with muscle and joint pain, missing the career and the life I'd once had, and terrified of what the future might hold. I was sad that my cherished teenaged sons were living five time zones, an eight-hour flight, and 4,913 miles away from me. I'd become all too aware of just how very alone and vulnerable I really was. So, within a space of five years, I'd transitioned from being a wildly healthy (or so I thought) young woman to a person whose body felt positively elderly. It was hard to feel like myself when my ego and almost every muscle in my body seemed to be waging war against the woman I'd once been.

By late 1990, my health was in a freefall. I'd moved to Florida because it reminded me (the sunshine, smiling faces, casual clothing, etc.) of the Los Angeles I had known as a college student. I was (again) uprooted, and worse, I could no longer walk. I officially and—very reluctantly—entered the dreaded, feared, and very challenging world of the disabled and wheelchair dependent.

At that point, I was still (at least) able to use both my hands. But it soon became obvious to me that the fingers on my right hand were no longer going to comply with my requests. Just as with my stubborn legs, it was a slow torturous type of downward progression, but the bottom line was that I couldn't brush my own hair, write legibly, type, or—scariest of all—needlepoint.

I'd begun needlepointing back in my early 20s, and it had become far more than just a hobby or crafting pastime to me. I loved the meditative sense of effortlessly watching small individual stitches get transformed into something beautiful. The normal dynamics of needlepointing (for a right-handed person like the pre-MS me) would be to hold the canvas in one's left hand, while a needle that contained one or two strands of Paternayan yarn is held between the thumb and index finger of the right hand.

Sadly, as the MS progressed, the fingers on my right hand refused to cooperate. I had grimly accepted the fact that my days of dancing and showjumping and walking were behind me, but I was determined to find a way to hold on to the one visually creative activity in my life that had always given me so much inspiration, solace, and satisfaction. Eventually, with the help of an adjustable wooden frame, I was able to tentatively teach myself how to adopt a different (and awkward) needlepoint technique that relied on the cooperation of my slow but still-functioning left hand.

A creative project that used to take me a month to complete, now requires half a year, but I like to tell myself that the finished product is still pleasing—in spite of the extra time it took. Perhaps being forced to use only my left hand (while in my 40s) was Mother Nature's way of making me embrace a slower, more laid-back, patient, and sanguine approach to my own definition of accomplishment and productivity.

While the honeybees use their entire bodies to create, harvest, and sculpt their beeswax honeycomb structures, I assemble thousands of tiny stitches with the help of my still-obedient left hand and a stiff wooden frame that sits on my lap. It took me several years to adapt to this new way of one-handed needlepointing, but the change has only enhanced the pleasure I still get from each completed gift item. What an amazing way to discover that Ludwig Mies van der Rohe (1886-1969) was presciently (for me) correct when he declared that *Less Is* [or can be] *More.*

WHAT THE HONEYBEES TAUGHT ME

- *Uncle Tom's Cabin* author, Harriet Beecher Stowe (1811-1896), might have been thinking of a beehive when she wrote, *"To be really great in little things, to be truly noble and heroic in the insipid details of everyday life, is a virtue so rare as to be worthy of canonization."*
- Small can still be spectacular.
- Not everything in life (or nature) can be replicated in a scientific laboratory.
- Legend has it that in 1910, Thomas A. Edison (1847-1931) invented the Honey Separator. Before that, people often ate honeycomb (which included traces of bee pollen and propolis) rather than "filtered" honey. Truly savvy beekeepers valued honeycomb that included Royal Jelly, Queen cells, and brood comb as well to their diet.
- Geometry—i.e., the academic study of shapes and sizes—is a honeybee's favorite form of math.
- With apologies to George Bernard Shaw (1856-1950), the Irish playwright who co-founded the London School of Economics, the beeswax and Royal Jelly-making worker bees teach us that sometimes *"Youth is* [not] *wasted on the young."*

Chapter 6
Honey

Kind words are like honey, sweet to the soul and healthy for the body.

Proverbs 16:24

Once I started getting bee stings, I began to stumble across a continually growing mountain of interesting historical tidbits about *Apis mellifera*. I learned that in Spain's *Cueve de la Arana* there is a 15,000 year old cave painting that depicts a woman gathering honey from a tree. And according to several paleontologists, bee fossils have been found that are estimated to be 150 million years old. And while there is no way to know whether or not honeybees existed during the Jurassic era, we do know that honey is mentioned in the Bible, the Koran and the Torah.

In long-ago Hindu wedding ceremonies, honey was traditionally applied to the bride's ears, eyelids, forehead, mouth, and genitals. Ancient Egyptian bridegrooms would use twelve jars of honey as a form of "commitment" to his bride, while their wedding guests would ingest honey-derived drinks for an entire month to celebrate the event. Beekeepers often enjoy telling enthusiastic newbies like me that the origin of "honeymoon" stems from the high regard that the Pharaohs had for honeybees and the sweetness they provided.

But my favorite historical honeybee story centers around a young Philadelphia beekeeper, who was a Quaker girl named Charity Crabtree. A Revolutionary soldier who had been wounded during a skirmish, begged her to deliver an important message to General George Washington. She jumped on her horse but realized that she would never be able to outrun the approaching British soldiers, so she came up with unique solution.

She knocked over the skeps that housed her honeybees, which resulted in the Redcoats being attacked and stung by the furious insects. Washington received the message, the British soldiers retreated, and Charity Crabtree was honored by our first President with these words; *"Neither you nor your bees shall be forgotten when our country is at peace again. It was the cackling geese that saved Rome, but it was the bees that saved America."*

***

For most of my life, I've been embarrassed by the fact that I have a massive sweet tooth. As a child, it was perfectly normal to prefer cookies and candy over more sensible food items, but as I grew older it began to seem not only immature, but irrational—if not blatantly unhealthy. I'd read books by Gayelord Hauser (1895-1984) when I was a teenager, which meant that (intellectually, at least) I knew the importance of vitamins and minerals. But (emotionally) I always chose the taste of something sweet over the healthier, nutrient-packed, and more sensible available option.

Almost 40 years ago, I met Sir Paul McCartney for an exclusive interview at his office—with its legendary massive Wurlitzer jukebox—in London. Within minutes of my arrival, a member of his staff set a tray down in front of us with coffee and "biscuits," which is the British term for cookies. I automatically, instinctively, and mindlessly reached for one, and was mortified when the former Beatle chuckled out loud. He'd laughed—endearingly—at the speed with which my fingers had lunged for the sweet calorie-laden carbohydrate in front of me. Even though he was charming and kind about my sugar-addicted child-like behavior, I still cringe at the memory of behaving like a naughty little girl with a sweet tooth, instead of a sensible journalist on an important assignment that was scheduled to be—after only one month on the paper—my first big front-page story.

The good news is that the potentially embarrassing day was saved when—just as I was packing up my notepad and tape recorder—Sir Paul thanked me for my time and kissed me on my right cheek. If, as a Beatles-crazy high school student in California, anyone had predicted that I would not only meet Paul McCartney, but have him hold my hand and give me a gentlemanly "goodbye" kiss, I probably would have died of cardiac arrest right on the spot.

The sense of discomfort that I'd always felt about preferring sweet over savory food items was recently assuaged when I learned that three different respected academics had made a surprising discovery point. They contributed to a unique research project titled "Sweet Taste Preferences and Experiences Predict Pro-Social Inferences, Personalities, and Behaviors." Their findings were published in the Journal of Personality and Social Psychology, and they indicate that individuals who prefer sweets tend to naturally be more agreeable and helpful, without necessarily being either more extroverted or neurotic. Evidently, thanks to this study, I no longer need to feel embarrassed about my irrational attachment to brownies, carrot cake, chocolate chip cookies, and peppermint bark...

***

Dr. Joel Fuhrman has written a number of best-selling books about the dangers of consuming "empty calories." And for decades, he's been heavily invested in the importance of maximizing the beneficial nutrients of what we eat as a way to optimize our health and longevity. But even though I am "knowledgeable" about and aware of what I should eat, I inevitably continue to prefer sweets over nutrients.

Long before I ever met him, I'd heard about the brilliant (now retired) board-certified neurologist, and Fellow of the American College of Nutrition, Dr. David Perlmutter, who is also a *New York Times* bestselling author. Dr. Perlmutter has made no secret of his disdain for sugar, and how it can compromise our health. While he acknowledges that humans' desire for sweets was actually "an early evolutionary advantage," he is saddened by the fact that over 65% of the foods sold in American grocery stores today include either added sugars or other artificial (i.e. chemical) sweeteners. The reason he is so against sugar is that research has revealed that it creates inflammation, which (among other drawbacks) is associated with the shrinking of brain tissue; and smaller brains contribute to an amped-up amygdala and poor decision-making.

According to several of the beekeepers I've interviewed, people who avoid honey because they feel it is as toxic as table sugar might benefit from investigating the topic a bit more. Technically, sugar is 50% fructose and 50% glucose, while honey is 40% fructose and 30% glucose. Honey's lower glucose content is why many diabetic patients can tolerate honey; essentially, less insulin is needed to metabolize its natural sugars.

Additionally, sugar is higher (100) on the Glycemic Index, while honey varies between 45 and 64, and that higher GI rating causes blood sugar levels to climb more quickly. In spite of that, however, one Tablespoon of sugar is only 49 calories, while the same amount of honey contains 64 calories. It's a sobering thought that during her entire six-week lifetime, a single bee will only be able to make less than a thimble-full of honey, which is less than a single Tablespoon.

For years, dentists have discouraged their patients from eating sugary foods because they lead to cavities. More recently, doctors are now concerned that sugar has a negative effect on the body's biome because it appears to reduce gut bacteria diversity. According to the American Heart Association women should consume no more than six teaspoons worth of sugar per day; men, however, can tolerate up to nine teaspoons.

If there were any question about honey's superiority over regular sugar, it could be settled by the fact that it has so many auxiliary nutrients (like beneficial enzymes), as well as by the fact that—as a natural source of a precursor to hydrogen peroxide—it can also be medically beneficial.

***

The enzymes in raw honey help the body digest it in a way that allows our system to process it without triggering a severe insulin reaction. Essentially, it's sweetness without a pancreatic stressor. One of my local experts recently told me that a Tablespoon of honey has the same "sweet effect" as an apple, and should be considered as an equivalent (and equally healthy) food choice. Honey contains small amounts of antioxidants, enzymes, pollen, protein, vitamins and minerals. And, depending on the source of the nectar that has been brought back to the hive, the honey will also contain a variety of both organic and amino acids.

Another misguided opinion about honey is that it is little more than "bee vomit." In truth, foraging bees have a special "crop" where they store the nectar they extract from flowers, and this internal storage area is separated from their other stomach with a valve that only works in one direction. So, if the honeybee needs additional energy while flying back home with the nectar, she can retrieve some of the nectar she's carrying without ever touching or being in contact with the contents of her "other" stomach. The returning foraging bee can store the pollen in one of her two stomachs, but the pollen is always kept isolated because bees have a small valve known as a "honey stopper" that keeps the contents of her two stomachs completely separated. During her entire six-week lifetime, a single bee will make less than a thimble full of honey.

***

Because honey contains so many beneficial trace elements, it would be wrong to assume that it is a totally harmless substance. In addition to the small number (three percent to five percent of the US population) of people who are severely allergic to bee venom, babies under the age of one should not eat honey. Ayurvedic practitioners argue that honey should not be included in hot beverages. Why? They believe that heat can release a toxin called hydroxymethel furfuraldehyde (HMF). Heat (even in baking) can change some of honey's chemical components, which can increase its peroxide levels. Ayurvedic doctors feel that heating honey makes it harder to digest because its components can develop an adhesive consistency. When that happens, the heat-altered honey sticks to the body's mucous membranes. This can make the detoxification process more difficult.

***

There are around 20,000 different types of bees in the world today, but only about 5% of them are the species that make honey, and those determined and hard-working mature honeybees usually visit 50 to 100 flowers during each collection trip. Statistically, a hive of bees will fly over 50,000 miles to produce a pound of honey, and in the course of a year a colony can produce anywhere from 60 to 100 pounds of honey. In other words, it takes the nectar from about two million different flowers to give us a single pound of golden honey.

A mature foraging worker bee drinks in as much watery nectar as she can, (somewhere in the neighborhood of about 400mg of nectar). That's about 0.0014 ounce, which is close to *one-third* of a honeybee's total body weight. After she flies back to the hive, she transfers the nectar to one of her waiting sisters. The young worker bees inside the hive help process what the foraging bees bring back. They are able to carry *twice* the amount of nectar (on their six legs) as the foraging bees that fly (using their four wings).

The fresh nectar that is brought back to the hive is about 80% water. "Finished honey," on the other hand, is only about 17% water. The young bee inside the hive that receives the nectar will hold the transferred liquid on her tongue until much of the water evaporates, and the nectar begins the process of becoming honey. At that point, it will be transferred into a hexagonal cell, aka, the honeycomb. This is the honey that will either be used by humans, or consumed by hungry worker bees when there is no "natural" nectar to be found. This transformation happens because the worker bees add enzymes and then "chew" the nectar until it is no longer thin and runny, and "dry" the mixture with their wings.

The transported nectar's resulting PH level (usually between 3.4 and 6.1) and low moisture level means that the honey can be stored for a very (very) long time. The process of turning nectar into honey is called "ripening," which happens in two stages. At first, the young bee sips nectar from the honeycomb cell and repeatedly rolls each droplet out to the tip of her tongue. This exposes it to air and begins the process of reducing the moisture content.

After about half of the nectar's water has evaporated, the droplet is returned to the honeycomb cell for the final stage of dehydration. This is accomplished when the bee fans her wings over the open honeycomb cells. Finally, after all the nectar has been deposited into the honeycomb cells, the honey then becomes "capped" with additional beeswax.

***

The South Florida beekeepers I've met introduced me to a different way of adding honey to my diet. Instead of just spreading honey on toast or adding it to sandwiches, these local experts make a habit of eating at least a teaspoon each day of fresh honeycomb. Sold in our local Farmers Markets for about $15, a four-inch square of honeycomb is an easy way to get all the benefits of honey, with the added bonus of small amounts of both pollen and propolis. They believe that chewing the honeycomb until all the honey is gone, and then swallowing the leftover wax is measurably beneficial for improved oral health. This practice can almost be considered a tasty form of Homeopathy because it contains trace elements of nutrients that benefit our teeth and gums.

One of my favorite local beekeepers—who has explored honeybee habits in the UK, Eastern Europe, and the US—warned me that his experiences with *Apis mellifera* was not at all what he had expected when he began his love affair with bees. With a chuckle, he confided—to paraphrase the popular Yorkshire author and veterinarian (whose real name was James Alfred Wight) James Herriot's (1916-1995) observation in *All Creatures Great and Small* — that the real problem areas were never the animals and wildlife. The problems, instead, came from people.

To illustrate his point, he told me, "If you get five beekeepers together and ask them a question about honeybees, I guarantee that you'll get six different very opinionated answers." As I continued with my own real-life bee research, I was relieved that I'd chosen to become "amateur enthusiast" rather than try to acquire an "expert" or "professional" status.

***

In 1865, an Austrian/Italian military leader named Franz Hruschka invented a machine that used centrifugal force to collect honey. Before that time, honeycomb had to be crushed by hand, which is why his invention is credited with transforming the modern honey industry. These days, when it's time to harvest honey, your local beekeeper probably uses a large stainless-steel drum-like device that can hold close to ten frames of honeycomb at a time. They will be suspended in wire baskets that are attached to the top of what is known as a "honey extractor." When the handle gets turned, a centrifugal force sends the honey flying out of the waxy cells of the honeycomb onto the machine's inside walls.

Some beekeepers insist that the sound the extractor's flywheel makes as it spins is actually similar to the hum of a beehive colony. The "released" honey then flows down the walls of the drum and—when it reaches the spigot—empty containers can (one at a time) easily be filled with honey one at a time. Small-scale beekeepers frequently wait to harvest their honey until the outdoor thermometer reads close to 90 degrees, because the heat makes the honey more liquid, and therefore more easy to work with.

Large-scale or professional beekeepers who have lots of hives can invest in electrically powered extractors that can actually hold more than 100 frames at a time. Before the frames—no matter how many—can be placed in the extractor, however, beekeepers need to use a long double-sided "uncapping" knife to scrape off the waxy seals at the top of each honeycomb cell.

As long as there is plenty of vegetation nearby, a honeybee can bring in several pounds of nectar in a single day. But if the nectar supply is even greater—and if there is lots of honeycomb in the hive to store it—foraging honeybees can bring back as much as ten pounds in a single (exhausting) day. According to one expert, it takes a dozen honeybees to gather enough raw nectar to produce just one teaspoon of honey; to do that, each of those mature bees needs to visit 2,500 flowers.

In a small-scale attempt to help the foraging bees, my friends and I have started planting bee-friendly bushes and flowers (Fuchsias seem to be their favorite) in our gardens. It has been estimated that the frequent trips back and forth from the pollen-rich flowers to the hive can be equal to the distance between Chicago and New York.

***

I am lucky to have easy access to clean, local, raw, unpasteurized honey because my good friend, Professor Vetaley Stashenko, has over 100 hives. He has become my go-to source for every hive product imaginable, from bee air to caps to eyedrops to propolis to pollen and Royal Jelly, as well as his four varieties of delicious local honey. But, until I became bee obsessed, I never realized that the honey sold in grocery stores, online, or even in health food stores could be suspect.

More than ever before, Americans love honey, and we've increased our consumption by 30% in only a decade. In 2019, we ate 1.69 pounds of honey per capita, which means that each and every one of us is consuming about 25 ounces per person. While that sounds like good news, it actually isn't. Why? Because American honey producers simply cannot generate that much on a consistent basis, so most of us are forced to eat large amounts of honey that has been imported from other less-regulated countries around the world. Sadly, the biggest importer is Asia, which is a part of the world that also has the least amount of guidelines regarding either the source purity or the processing techniques.

That's why—each year—we import about half a million metric tons of honey from China, 117,000 metric tons from Turkey, 79,000 from Iran, 78,000 from Argentina, and 69,000 from Ukraine. While much of this less-desirable imported honey is sold to the food conglomerates commercially, a great deal of it still winds up in our own kitchens.

Sadly, far too much of the (less-costly) honey currently made available to American consumers has been diluted with high fructose corn syrup, maltose syrup, "ultra-filtered" honey, and a variety of other unhealthy products that—to those of us who are passionate about the subject—is little more than a poor but (affordable) excuse for honey. As usual, the advice *Caveat Emptor* (Buyer Beware) is worth remembering.

***

My first happy memory of falling in love with the taste of honey began with my childhood Saturday morning breakfasts in the 1950s, when my *uber*-housewife mother would invariably make homemade buttermilk biscuits. Long before I was allowed to handle a knife by myself, she would mix a large pat of butter (as a teenager I replaced it with peanut butter) into a generous serving of honey, and then spread the mixture on an opened steaming-hot biscuit fresh from the oven. As a little girl, it was my idea of culinary nirvana, and—when it comes to my hard-wired taste preferences—during the ensuing half century, very little has changed.

It took working on this book for me to understand how I developed my life-long sweet tooth. I grew up in a family that always—every single night—ended our dinner with some sort of homemade desert. My mother frequently made a wide variety of pies, but her Pineapple Upside Down, Coconut, and Carrot cakes were simply wonderful. Long before I was able to enroll in Kindergarten, I'd learned that there would always be something sweet to "reward" me for eating other foods (like animal protein and dark green leafy vegetables) that I simply didn't particularly like.

As the years progressed and life got increasingly stressful, I searched frantically to find tasty little "rewards" wherever I could. Most often, they arrived either in the form of colorful fresh fruits, inside a Lindt or See's chocolate shop, a bakery item in a pink cardboard box, or fresh homemade creations that came out of my own cinnamon-scented oven.

I knew only too well how everyone from Adelle Davis (1904-1974) and Dave Asprey and Dr. Steven Gundry and Dr. Mark Hyman, and all the other health writers I've admired feel about sugar-filled foods. But by the time I'd turned 30, it was clear to me that a well-prepared chocolate *ganache* would always hold far more appeal to me than any dinner entree from a Michelin-starred restaurant ever would. Having MS has altered every aspect of my life—from my strength to my confidence level to my sense of humor—but it hasn't diminished my taste buds' need for sweets.

What a relief—as a still-evolving health-conscious Senior Citizen—to have finally discovered good, clean, natural honey as the ultimate guilt-free source of sweetness. Perhaps, for the first time ever, with the help of local beekeepers, I will soon be able to simultaneously nourish my body and "reward" my sugar-addicted psyche as I continue the struggle to get healthier. Who could possibly ask for anything more?

WHAT THE HONEYBEES TAUGHT ME

- One small pound of honey is the result of nectar that has been collected from (literally) millions of flowers and has traveled as much as 40,000 miles (that's more than one trip around the globe). Mature foraging bees will easily fly up to three miles away from their hives as they relentlessly search for nectar and pollen and propolis.

- Honey is the ultimate—and perhaps only—eco-friendly sweetener. Sugars derived from beets, corn, and sugar cane have a large carbon footprint, but honey doesn't require challenging human labor to harvest, the use of toxic fertilizers, harmful pesticides, more costly irrigation systems.

- In the US alone, there are over 300 varieties of honey, but (as with wine) honey is never exactly the same from harvest to harvest, season to season, or year to year. Some honey aficionados, however, insist that the darker a honey's color, is the more nutrients (antioxidants, pollen, vitamins, minerals, etc.) it will probably have.

- It only takes one ounce of harvested honey to fuel a bee's flight all the way around the globe, not that she would ever want to willingly go that far away from her own hive.

- In ancient Hindu (Sanskrit) writings, the word *Madhukara* often has three meanings: bee, lover, and moon. It is considered to be the origin of the word "honeymoon."

- In 1694, when German Botanist Rudolph Jakob Camerarius (1665-1721) first published his theory on plant pollination, it was considered "obscene." Decades later, Philip Miller (1691-1771) described honeybees extracting nectar from tulip flowers, but his observations were also considered "distasteful." In fact, in the mid-1700s, the third, fourth, and fifth, editions of *The Gardener's Dictionary* was forced to delete any mention of honeybee pollination because it was considered too racy. Wow, have times and values ever changed?!

Chapter 7
Physiology

Whatever happens to your body, your soul will survive, untouched.

HARRY POTTER AND THE DEATHLY HALLOWS
J.K. Rowling

I chose the above quote for two very personal reasons. First, having held the hands of loved ones on their deathbed, I do believe that the body and the soul are separate entities, and both need to be assiduously cared for and treasured. The other reason, is because J.K. Rowling's mother (like me) had MS. I like to think that this wrenching experience gave Britain's most successful author an added dollop of compassion and sensitivity regarding what our bodies can, should, and cannot do.

After I met Michael and his bees, I read Pat Wagner's 1994 book (*How Well Are You Willing To Bee?)* about her astonishing journey from being bed ridden with MS to regaining her mobility. I had been deeply impressed by the fact that–once her health had been restored–she generously reached out and helped others by offering bee stings at her suburban home. Learning about her journey, propelled me to an even greater sense of chronic Stubborn Optimism.

After only two months (eight sessions) of bee stings (otherwise known as bee venom therapy or BVT), I began to get internal whispered hints that—

both emotionally and physically—good things were beginning to happen. Michael had told me from the very beginning of our "experiment" that this would be a long, slow, but ultimately health-enhancing and beneficial procedure. The bee stings were part of a natural process of trying to rebuild my health on a cellular level, which could take years instead of months. In the past, I'd often been called the most impatient woman on planet Earth, but when it came time to work with the honeybees and their venom, I'd waited so long (and so desperately) that I was more than willing to—if necessary—wait, and wait, and then even wait some more.

During my first five or ten sting sessions, by the time Michael packed up his remaining bees, I definitely felt physically beat-up. It was a short-lived general feeling—similar to having an annoying case of the flu—that would find me alternating between a mild fever, light chills, and a complete loss of appetite. I would usually nap for an hour or two after receiving close to a dozen stings, but with each session, the symptoms seemed less and less irritating or unpleasant. The sting sites would often be itchy at first, but I actually began to sense a gentle post-sting feeling of inner cleansing and clarity, which I'd never experienced before.

The next physical change that I noticed— almost immediately—was that my fingernails regained the strength and shape they'd had before my MS diagnosis. Until MS began its aggressive attempt to take over my body, my health, and my life, I'd always had very long rock-hard fingernails that rarely broke, and never split or peeled. So, I was delighted to see that my former fingernail health had returned so quickly once the honeybees began to sting me every week. Michael, however, was not at all surprised by the improvement.

I'll be the first to admit that when I shared news flashes about the first handful of small physical changes I'd observed, they were far from being earth-shattering improvements. But when you've lived with MS for over 30 years, and if during that time everything you've ever heard or experienced about your body's wellbeing is depressing, discouraging, or painful, it makes perfect sense to celebrate even the most minute positive development. And heaven knows, after adapting to the pain and itching of the beestings, I was definitely in the mood to celebrate anything and everything I could.

Ramon, my delightfully observant caregiver, actually pointed out the next subtle change that (again) was minor, but definitely measurable. Each morning, Ramon has a set schedule that he follows to help me get ready to greet the day. Once he arrives at my home, and after he helps me get to the bathroom so I can brush my teeth, Ramon does his best to make me as presentable as possible; part of that process includes brushing my hair. After I had been getting stung for about six weeks, he pointed out that there were a lot fewer hairs left in my brush than there had been before the honeybees became part of our regular routine. Again, when I mentioned this to Michael, he was not at all surprised.

As I mentioned earlier, Michael had experienced a "bee healing" event of his own years ago, and he makes no secret of the fact that he truly believes bee venom therapy (BVT) acts as a booster or stimulant for our body's individual and unique immune system. He'd already warned me that major muscular advances would take a very long time, but smaller signs of "baby-step improvements" would continue to gradually and sporadically appear. I was beginning to learn that just as honeybees have their own sense of timing for accomplishment and productivity, our recuperating bodies heal by following their own very individualized concept of time.

***

While an active hive might look as if it is run by robot workers, a honeybee hive is actually a complex grouping of individuals. Most beekeepers openly respect and intellectually admire the honeybees' inherent ability to communicate, memorize, and make decisions. Honeybees even have the ability to "solve" specific and unique problems. One example of this ability is that honeybees in Asia have kept Killer Hornets away from their nests and hives by spreading malodorous feces at the entrance to their homes. *Apis mellifera* are obsessive about cleanliness within their own domiciles, but they've found a brilliant (if icky) way to repel attackers and protect their family.

Honeybees—with their four fragile wings, five buggy eyes, six useful legs, and large antenna—really do look like a prototypical insect. The standard adult worker bee has a body that's divided into three parts: head, thorax, and abdomen. Very young developing bees, however, actually wiggle (and look like) translucent maggots.

Essentially, the **head** helps the honeybee process information, and it contains antenna, eyes, and mouth. The first third of a worker bee's body contains everything she needs in order to eat, navigate, see, smell, and gather things like pollen or propolis. Honeybees have surround-sound ultraviolet vision, interconnected wings, as well as antenna that can detect movement and odor to identify everything from explosives to cancers to flowers.

Apis Mellifera's antenna are two L-shaped sticks that swivel in their sockets. There are five different eyes on a honeybee's forehead, and the large ones are like two black shiny commas. A honeybee can "translate" ambient sounds and vibration by using their antennas, their antennas' short hairs and small pegs, which respond to air movement, temperature, and water content. The antennas are also able to measure the depth of various flower petals. And when it comes to the bees' nest (or hive)—where there is very little (if any) available light—honeybees also use their antenna to find each other and share information from various sources within the hive.

A bee's antenna actually affects its body while in flight because it appears to react to the earth's magnetic field. And since flowers give off a gentle electromagnetic charge, the antenna (which are only two millimeters apart) can easily pick up their message. They can also detect fragrance, which is handy when hunting for nectar.

Honeybees have what is called "Ocelli," which are three light sensors that live above their two large eyes. The two large eyes are compound, while the other three have thousands of facets. Each one of those facets has its own lens and sensory cells that help the bee recognize colors, light, and patterns. People used to think that bees were colorblind, but in fact their eyes simply register color differently than ours do. To a foraging honeybee, green actually looks gray, and red appears black. And while our human eyes do not register colors at the ultraviolet end of the spectrum, bees easily see those hues.

Honeybees' five furry eyeballs are particularly gifted at picking up ultraviolet light. Worker bees rely on the location of the sun to help them navigate, but even on cloudy days their ability to "translate" ultraviolet rays allows them to operate with their own very effective GPS system. Some researchers believe that honeybees somehow have enough brainpower (in the size of a sesame seed) to coordinate and direct the movement of their twelve separate appendages.

Drones who need to be able to identify a virgin Queen in flight have over 8,000 facets in each of their compound eyes. Worker bees don't need to have such exacting vision, so they only have about 6,000 facets per eye. The Queen, who spends almost all of her life at home, in the dark, laying thousands of eggs each day, has only 3,000 to 4,000 facets in her eyes.

Human eyes don't have facets; instead, we have lenses.

A bee's tongue is actually shaped like a straw, which allows her to suck nectar from the base of the flowers she visits. On both sides of her head, she has mandibles, which are like jaws that help her chew honey or pollen, and shape wax.

The **thorax**, which is behind the head, helps a honeybee move to where it needs to go. The thorax is like a large hard-shelled muscle that has built-in attachments for a honeybee's six legs and four wings. Those legs have tiny hooks on their feet, and they can use their first four legs to stroke and groom their antenna or grasp small items. A honeybee's exterior orange bands also have tiny hairs, and the black hairs are actually slick. The way to gauge the actual age of a honeybee is to look for golden "baby down" on its thorax.

Within the thorax, bees have a very long esophagus. A honeybee's thorax has three sections, and each one has its own pair of legs. Additionally, the last two sections also have one pair of wings each—the front set of wings has a fold that runs along the outer edge, while the back pair of wings have tiny barbs that can hook onto the fold of the front wings (almost like Velcro). This can come in handy if the foraging bee needs one larger set of strong wings instead of two smaller less powerful ones.

While Drones and Queens do not have pollen or propolis gathering leg capabilities, all worker bees have front legs that include a specific type of brush mechanism that allows them to clean their antenna and scoop up any loose pollen.

After the thorax, the body becomes a bit slimmer, and beneath the waist her **abdomen** holds the working organs and mechanisms needed for fluid circulation, breathing, and food digestion. A honeybee's abdomen is home to all its vital organs; the last one is its stinger, which delivers bee venom.

The abdomen is where the honeybees' specific glands are located. Some are for smell, some are to make wax, plus there is the poison gland that creates bee venom. The honeybees' abdomen includes its heart, and the circulatory systems for *haemolynph* (bee blood), as well as the honey stomach and its true (separate) stomach. Bees also have small holes (spiracles) that provide air to the trachea and the inside air sacs of the honeybee's body.

Neither the Queen nor the drones have a Nasanov gland, which is a shiny light brown bulge near one of a worker bees' stripes. This tiny gland produces a lemongrass-like scent that can be used by bees to mark a particular territory. Spreading this scent near the hive entrance helps other family members find their way back home.

Most foraging bees leave the hive around thirteen times each day in search of nectar, and they will typically visit 100 flowers each trip. Foraging bees will have worn away that fuzz while searching for nectar. A foraging bee sometimes gets her entire body dusted with pollen after she's been nectar hunting, and this activity will soon wear away her "fuzz." She will move much of that valuable powder into the "baskets" that are on her hind legs, and this is how she takes the pollen back to the hive where it will be used as food for developing larvae. At the end of a bee's legs are "miniature feet" that can find cracks in otherwise smooth surfaces. They are similar to a cat's nails, and are called "tarsal claws."

The largest bee in a hive is, of course, the Queen. But each hive also has a small number of drones, who are almost twice the size of an ordinary worker bee. Drones have larger eyes and a more square-shaped body than the worker bees; they do not, however, have a stinger.

***

According to a research consortium supported by the National Human Genome Research Institute (NHGRI), the western honeybee's genome is more similar to human beings to any other insect's sequence so far. While the honeybee's genome is only nine percent of the size of the three billion base pairs of the human genome, it contains almost half as many genes as the human genome. In other words, humans have around 20,000 genes, while honeybees have more than 10,000. I took this "connection" as a reason to further explore the myriad ways that MS had hijacked my health.

At first, I thought about comparing the strengths and weaknesses of my own body with that of the industrious worker bee. But when I realized that my battle with MS would (literally) never exist within the bee community, I understood that I needed to stop hunting for hidden similarities, and accept the fact that my MS battle would be something that the group-conscious community of industrious worker bees would never accept or condone or tolerate. In the honeybee world, anything or anyone that might compromise the wellbeing of the other bees is automatically scheduled for immediate execution. It is a self-protective *Apis mellifera* mechanism that allows the hive to remain productive without getting sidetracked or distracted by the individual needs of an ill or injured family member.

In the past, I've avoided writing about my physical MS struggles because I felt awkward about sharing my private challenges with the world at large. More than most, I know how unfair it is to expect healthy able-bodied people to understand what it's like to go through life unable to accomplish the simplest of tasks without (a million times a day) asking someone else for assistance.

There are a handful of individuals in my life who have had an honest glimpse of what it's like to live inside my compromised and uncooperative body. But for the majority of people with whom I come in contact, I have done my best to keep my physical pain as well as my frustrations and medical problems under wraps. Part of the reason is discretion, part of the reason is my ego-driven need to not be pitied, and part is that I truly want to shield them from witnessing my unappealing private struggles.

As I've mentioned before, every case of MS is different, which means that while I can tell you about some of my particular symptoms, I cannot speak for others who are members of this exceptionally cruel club. In an earlier chapter, I shared how Dr. David Perlmutter who (like many neurologists) was surprised to discover that an overgrowth of bad intestinal bacteria is the root cause of most neurological complications. When I first read his theory, it triggered a memory of a strange pre-diagnosis event back in 1984 when I had a bizarre sensation that made no sense at all at the time—but now it does.

As usual, on the night in question, I'd returned home from an exhausting day at the *Los Angeles Times,* and had enjoyed a quiet evening with my two sons. By 10 p.m., they were both asleep in their rooms, and I was alone in my king-sized bed surrounded with books and papers that needed my attention before I returned to the office first thing in the morning. A close girlfriend called to inquire about my plans for the upcoming weekend, and after we'd coordinated our Saturday schedules, I told her that I was experiencing an unusual abdominal sensation.

"Honestly," I told her, *"it feels as if I'm wearing control-top pantyhose that are too tight. It's almost as if that part of my body is tingling."*

"Well, maybe you should take off your pantyhose," she replied with a chuckle.

When I told her that I'd changed into my nightgown hours earlier, and was just lying in bed waiting to go to sleep—with no pantyhose (control-top or otherwise) on. She then admitted that she'd never heard of a 10 p.m. case of an unusual "vibrating" abdomen. The strange feeling gradually went away, and I didn't think anything more about it until I read Dr. Perlmutter's book, which let me know that almost 40 years earlier I'd experienced my first MS symptom, which is now referred to as "leaky gut syndrome."

***

Honeybees actually have their own unique language, and they have been known to sing when happy, shriek when scared, growl angrily when they are threatened, and be mute when they are sad. The Queen Bee is able to make a specific sound (often thought of as a war cry) when she is threatened. When it comes to sound inside the hive, researchers claim that the adult bees generate 190 vibrations per second. For the musically inclined, that would be represented by a note halfway between F# and G, and below middle C on the piano. When the foraging honeybees fly, the vibrations increase to 248 per second, which would be the sound of B.

Here in South Florida, it's sunny and warm most of the year. But in areas where there are four distinct seasons, a beehive in winter can sound much different from one in summer. When it's warm, the beehive will include thousands of adult female worker bees, lots of young female workers, a small number of male drones, and lots of workers of all ages perusing their different jobs, and creating unique sounds. But in cold weather, the drones—who contributed nothing to the hive community while they waited for a new virginal Queen they could impregnate—are enthusiastically executed by the fed-up and fatigued worker bees.

Newly-hatched female larvae already have adult-sized bodies, but their wings don't become hard enough to support flight until they are at least nine days old. When these "youngsters" do flap their fragile wings (for either ventilation or warming purposely inside the hive) their wings are able to move faster than the adults'. As a result, their activity creates a higher audible sound. The drones, on the other hand, have larger wings that move more slowly and have a lower note. Here is a list of the most common honeybee notes. (# signifies sharp.)

- Very young bee fanning her wings C#-D
- Six day old bee fanning her wings A-A#
- Adult worker bee fanning her wings F#-G
- Adult worker bee flying B
- Adult guard bee in attack mode C-C#
- Drone flying flat low C

Honeybees in Asia have recently been observed creating a unique noise with their wings that researchers describe as an "anti-predator pipe" (otherwise known as a bee scream). These bees only make this specific noise when they have been threatened by Killer Hornets that are approaching their hives or nests.

Honeybees are so particular about the cleanliness of their homes that during cold weather, they don't defecate until the weather is warm enough for them to go out outside. Beekeepers who live in colder climates often witness the bees' "cleansing flights." This is when the bees use the first sign of warm weather to (finally) leave the hive and frantically "relieve themselves" by depositing what looks like splattered yellow egg yolk "poop" as quickly as possible after waiting so long.

***

Although I'd dealt with a limp and some numbness before my symptoms went into remission, after I moved to London, it felt as if my health took a pretty severe nosedive. I was still hoping that a more benign reason than MS was at the root of my walking challenges, but when the next symptom appeared it felt like a massive and ominous red flag had just been unfurled directly above my head.

I was seated at my desk at *The Daily Mail*, where I was surrounded with what felt like a sea of balding, smoking, much-older hardened male journalists who viewed me—as the new-hire, young female author imported from *Los Angles Times*—with undisguised skepticism. I loved my new job, which required me to keep my passport in my purse at all times just in case my editor decided to send me ASAP—to Paris or New York or Buenos Aires or Hollywood in order to snag a high-profile celebrity interview. That was the fun, exciting part of my life at that time.

What wasn't fun was the realization that I had uprooted my sons, left my large, friendship heavy support system, and done so with the shadow of a serious (ignored but undeniable) shadow of a degenerative disease always in the background.

Fueled by my Stubborn Optimism, I had hoped so fervently for the best possible scenario that I'd never taken the time to come face-to-face with what just might turn into the worst probable outcome.

An event that truly frightened me happened when(six months into my five-year stay in London)I was seated at my metal newsroom desk, which (in the pre-computer days when seasoned British journalists still used manual typewriters) held the only electric typewriter on the floor. On an otherwise ordinary morning I tried to do something that I'd—reflexively and unconsciously—done millions of times before. In the middle of the noisy room, with reporters and photographers passing by my desk on a regular basis, I began to research the latest celebrity I was due to interview for the next day. I was scheduled to meet Jackie Collins at the Ritz Hotel in Piccadilly to discuss the film adaptation of her latest best-selling book, and I had all the paperwork regarding her life story spread out before me.

Just before I took a sip of my coffee, I decided to cross my legs to get just a bit more comfortable in my chair. I was shocked and terrified to discover that—at that moment—there was no way I could persuade my right leg to cross over my left knee. No matter how urgently my thoughts directed my leg to move, my right foot stubbornly remained on the floor.

All around me, it was just another busy morning at a London newspaper office, but I had the sinking premonition that my life—from that moment onward—was probably going to be dramatically different from anything I had ever imagined or known before. Sadly, I was 100% correct.

WHAT THE HONEYBEES TAUGHT ME

- The French author Colette (1873-1954) probably wasn't thinking about honeybees when she made this observation: *Our perfect companions never have fewer than four feet,* but she could have been...
- Honeybees are compulsive about doing their jobs, and doing them well; they have no idea what fatigue or self-pity, or sorrow is, and they never ever give up.
- Both humans and honeybees are closely connected to our Circadian Rhythm, which affects everything for us and for them—from appetite to communication and sleep patterns.
- Honeybees are not equipped to identify with or care about the less fortunate. But anthropologist Margaret Mead(1901-1978) would have said that the insect world is too primitive for compassion. In her words, *"Helping someone else through difficulty is the starting point of civilization."* She also observed *"Never doubt that a small group of thoughtful, committed citizens can change the world; for, indeed, that's all who ever have."*
- Knowing what I now know about honeybees, Christopher Robin's advice to Winnie the Pooh (*"Always remember you are braver than you believe, smarter than you seem, and stronger than you think."*) could have been directed at those tiny little worker bees who spend their short lifespan making our lives so much better.

Chapter 8
Urban Honeybees

I want to wake up in a city that doesn't sleep.

NEW YORK, NEW YORK,
Fred Ebb (1928-2004) and John Kander

I love the fact that no matter how old we get, life still contains plenty of surprises. And if you were lucky enough to have been born under a lucky star—like me—many of those unexpected developments turn out to be delightful ones. As 2020 began—just before COVID-19 hijacked our lives—I began to sense some surprising emotional and physical shifts that signaled the positive impact that the bee venom was having on my life.

After I'd had weekly bee sting sessions for about six months, I began to notice positive changes that were less subtle than the ones I'd already tracked. While the first noticeable changes had been largely superficial (hair, nails, etc.), after I'd had about 25 visits from Michael and his bees, bigger improvements slowly began to surface.

It's not as if I miraculously regained my mobility, or that my limbs began to obey me whenever I asked them to move. Instead, the overall feeling of wellbeing kept inching upwards. As with so many things about "Bee Healing," the changes were subtle and almost indescribable, but I could feel—internally—that something positive was happening. The closest way I can describe this unusual sensation would be to recall a 1981 cartoon commercial for a household cleaning product. According to the ad, small "Scrubbing Bubbles" were guaranteed to restore cleanliness and vibrancy no matter how soiled the stubborn area in question might be.

Intellectually, I'm not comfortable with comparing what was going on inside my body with a chemical household cleaner, but emotionally that's exactly how my body felt. Nothing that I have heard or read or watched has ever referred to bee venom as a natural cleansing product, but since every MS patient has a unique set of circumstances, for now I'll just stick with mine.

By December of 2019, I was pleasantly surprised to sense a slowly-growing feeling of increased muscular strength in my left arm and hand, instead of the ever-present "floppy feeling" that MS had brought my way so many years before. One aspect of having MS that very few people have written about is the emotional impact of dealing with an uncooperative body. Both pain and paralysis present their own levels of difficulty, but for me, coping with a million little emotionally frustrating challenges proved far more painful than dealing with sheer physical discomfort.

One of those reoccurring frustrations was the fact that only being able to use my (sporadically unreliable) left hand meant that way, way, way too often I would either drop items or knock them over (books, food, glasses, papers, etc.). For an able-bodied person this would just be an accidental, two-second non-event, but for me it represented that I had—yet again—(a) created a mess, (b) frequently broken an item, and now needed someone else's help to (c) retrieve said item, and then (d) clean up whatever had been knocked over or spilled. Each time that happened it served as a crushing reminder that (according to the doctors) I would be increasingly dependent on other people's assistance for the rest of my life. A wiser more serene woman would have probably shrugged off those silly annoyances, but for me, every dropped item triggered a new wave of annoyance, fear, frustration and sadness, and (all too frequently) tears.

Imagine my surprise when, after receiving about 500 bee stings, it dawned on me that I actually hadn't dropped or knocked anything over for weeks. As I've mentioned before in this book, when it comes to honeybees, I have never thought of myself as an expert. I'm not an academic, I'm not a professional beekeeper, and my brain has very few (if any) scholarly scientific synapses.

But there was no way that I could ignore the inexplicable connection between the additional bee stings and the elimination of an annoying and repetitive problem that had grown gradually worse over three very challenging decades. Again, when I told Michael about my "discovery," he was pleased but not at all surprised.

There was no way that the next change could be considered "imaginary" or "wishful thinking," because it was witnessed (and acknowledged) by others. Ever since 2006, I had been lucky enough to receive weekly occupational and physical therapy sessions at the Rehabilitation Center for Children and Adults (RCCA) in Palm Beach. Since I am unable to move three of my four extremities, this means that my spectacular occupational therapist, Kelli Jacobs, struggles every Monday morning to move my arms and legs. Her skill and training helps them stay as supple and strong as possible—given the situation. Kelli is too professional (and far too kind) to ever complain about the sheer effort it takes to fight the creeping stiffness of MS, but I know that our sessions can be physically taxing for her.

When we first began working together, our sessions would easily "lose" about 15 minutes each time because—without warning—my uncooperative legs would develop spasms. My right leg in particular would feel like a massive Charley Horse to me, but it must've seemed like an unmovable slab of concrete for Kelli. Those spasms complicated her efforts to bend my knees, flex my ankles, or twist my hips. It was only a matter of months into my "bee venom experiment" before Kelli and I both noticed that our sessions were no longer being interrupted by uncomfortable (and unwelcome) muscle spasms. As a result, Kelli began introducing additional stretches and strengthening movements that would have been unthinkable back when my MS-stiffened body was doing everything possible to thwart her hands-on-therapeutic technique.

I also cherished my weekly two hours at RCCA because that's where I was able to use the stationary

NuStep bicycle. This piece of equipment is ideal for paraplegics and people with MS because it allows us to get a mild cardio workout thanks to the involvement of all four limbs. When I first became an RCCA patient, I wasn't considered a candidate to use the NuStep bike, but I pestered and pleaded with physical therapist extraordinaire Ellen O'Bannon so persistently that she finally agreed to let me "try" the bike to see how I would fare.

The bike has adjustable controls, with one-to-ten difficulty levels, and it can track how many "steps" per minute a user has made. With my right hand inside a glove that was velcroed to the handlebar, and both my feet strapped to the pedals, on my first session I was able to complete five minutes at level one. Today, 17 years later, I routinely complete 15-to-20 minutes at level six. In light of the fact that— according to the experts—MS patients never improve, this is one of my proudest "athletic" achievements ever. Naturally, Michael was pleased, but not at all surprised...

Just as with the end of randomly-dropped items, there was no way for me to "verify" that my physical improvements were related to the bee venom. Still, nothing else in my life that could have affected my muscles (diet, lifestyle, etc.) had changed. My Stubborn Optimism assured me that something about the bee sessions was definitely having a positive effect on various aspect of my health. I was only too aware of the fact that—each time I would enthusiastically announce that something (anything) was improving instead of declining—a number of people in my life would ever-so-subtly roll their eyes, then nod indulgently, and congratulate me on my "Positive Attitude." No one wanted to burst my hope-filled balloon, but they were also skeptical about such an esoteric and offbeat (not to mention painful) regimen.

***

Do you remember the Aesop fable *The Town Mouse and the Country Mouse*? While I never totally identified with either the country bumpkin or the smooth city slicker, the disparity between small-town security and big-city excitement has always occupied a major portion of my consciousness. After all, my youth was spent relocating from one small town (*Manhattan Beach, Newport, Toledo, Yuma, etc.*) to another. Until I enrolled at UCLA, my only experience of living in the middle of a big city came via books, magazines, movies, newspapers, and TV shows. It didn't take long, however, for me to turn into (practically overnight) a concrete flower who preferred sidewalks and freeways to small towns and country roads.

***

While many of us imagine a clump of white wooden beehives nestled on a grassy hillside in the country, in reality, big-city rooftop honeybee communities are growing as never before. Of late, many experts have been surprised to see the 21st century explosion of big-city beekeeping. Once metropolitan areas became aware of the value of crosspollination (close to 90% of flowering plants and wildflowers, as well as 75% of fruits, nuts, and vegetables in the American diet, benefit from visits by honeybees), they stopped restricting beehives within city limits.

Today, Boston, Chicago, Detroit, Miami, New York City, Philadelphia, San Francisco, and Washington DC, are among the many major American cities that welcome Urban Beekeeping.

Internationally, Amsterdam, Berlin, Brussels, Frankfurt, Hamburg, Hong Kong, Istanbul, Johannesburg, London, Melbourne, Montevideo, Paris, Santiago, Singapore, Sydney, Tokyo, Toronto, Utrecht, and Vancouver have also begun welcoming the urban honeybee movement. My favorite city, London, has more than doubled the number of registered beehives during the last ten years, and currently has 7,500 rooftop beehives. As of this writing, London is believed to have the densest honeybee population of any European city. In London, Bermondsey Street Bees actually uses the Royal Botanic Garden's Kew Gardens map to determine and pinpoint beehive density. What has now been labeled "an Urban renaissance in apiculture," is particularly popular in Europe. For example, in only six years (between 2006 and 2012) the number of beekeepers in Berlin grew by over 50%.

Many experts have been surprised that big-city honeybee colonies actually appear to be stronger and more productive than some of their "country cousins." At first, it was assumed that this advantage was the result of the honeybees being less exposed to crop fertilizers, and the particularly toxic neonicotinoid agricultural pesticides. Non-lethal exposure to these poisons damage a bee's ability to return to her hive after foraging for nectar. Sadly, this chemically-induced confusion winds up having a negative effect on the entire population of a honeybee community. For this reason, the European Union is debating whether to ban (or severely restrict) the use of neonicotinoid pesticides. But another equally important factor may also be at work...

According to the USDA, more than 50% of American cropland is devoted to mono-culture crops (particularly corn and soybean), which limits a honeybee's diet diversity. Bees that forage for "polyfloral pollen" appear to have stronger immune systems and longer survival rates than honeybees that are only able to retrieve one specific type of pollen.

The *Apis mellifera* that are part of the growing urban beekeeping movement appear to be measurably healthier simply because of the nectar and pollen diversity that is available within large city spaces. While it may be hard to imagine, thousands of honeybees living happily on a skyscraper roof is exactly what is happening all over the globe. In Manhattan, hives can be found on top of the Brooks Brothers Flagship, as well as InterContinental New York Barclay Hotel, and the New York Institute of Technology. For years, the Waldorf Astoria Hotel has provided honey for its chefs, residents, and visitors.

And Boston's Museum of Science has a "Best Bees'" hive that helps younger children learn about the importance of honeybees. Kitchen garden bees can also be found atop Manhattan's Sofitel, and even at the White House (where in only four years over 175 pounds of honey was harvested).

**

I first became aware of the urban beekeeper movement when I watched a TED Talk and a Netflix documentary about the importance of honeybees. Thanks to those videos I learned about Fulbright Scholar Andrew Coté, a fourth-generation beekeeper who is also the president of the New York City Beekeepers Association. He sells "Andrew's Honey" at Manhattan's Union Square Green Market and is the executive director of Bees Without Boarders. Up until about a decade ago, it was (yikes!) illegal to keep bees in New York City, but Coté and his colleagues have managed to make rooftop beehives a reality on iconic buildings like the Museum of Modern Art and United Nations.

When I read Coté's book (*Honey and Venom: Confessions of an Urban Beekeeper*), I learned about his international honeybee travels with his father. Their goal has been to teach beekeepers how to harvest more honey and protect the bees in far-flung locales like China, Ecuador, Fiji, Iraq, and Uganda.

In New York City today, there are (officially) over 300 rooftop hives. Andrew Coté, however, believes that the number within New York's city limits is closer to 600. I in Paris, there are actually over 2,000. As is often the case, the rise of city beekeeping means that honeybee-protective companies have emerged to help well-meaning amateurs. In addition to Boston's "Best Bees," there's also the Montreal company "Alvéole," Long Island's "Promised Land Apiaries," and "Beacon Partners," which has hives on top of 25 American buildings, and plans to add another dozen rooftop hives soon. And even though much of the honey used for their wide variety of products comes from rural plants, *Bees in the D*, has placed a growing number of hives on building rooftops in Detroit.

"Apiterra" is an urban beekeeping firm that cares for over 300 hives scattered across Paris (L'Oréal, AXA, and the Saint-Germain football club, are among its clients). Also in Paris, a company named "Beeopic" cares for 350 hives located on top of the Grand Palais Hall, BNP Paribas SA, and LVMH. In 2021, "Beeopic" was acquired by Montreal's "Avéole," which cares for over 3,000 beehives at 600 different companies in 20 North American cities. Back in 2010, there were only 300 registered beehives in Paris, but now that number is fast approaching 3,000.

Avéole charges around $2,000 per hive per year, and clients have the opportunity to participate in candle-making classes and honey production instruction. The company was founded back in 2013 by three environmentally-motivated McGill University graduates.

One unexpected advantage of urban beekeeping is that the big city honeybee colonies seem to survive better during cold-weather months than their rural counterparts. In exchange, the bees help keep the city landscape green, well pollinated, and they offer a small solution to the chronic problem of CCD (colony collapse disorder).

One potential problem for urban beekeepers, however, is that some cities (like Berlin, London, and Paris) now have beehive concentrations as high as 20 hives for every square kilometer of land. As a result, the honeybees are forced to compete with bumblebees, butterflies, and wild (or feral) bees for available nectar and pollen. That helps explain why Boston's "The Best Bees Company" evaluates local honey in over a dozen US cities to measure the quality of pollen available to local honeybees.

British-based "Green Roof Organization" has followed a program developed in the Netherlands to plant sedum (a hearty plant that resists drought and is pollinator friendly) at city bus stops. These planted areas are now referred to as "bee bus stops" and are currently part of the Leicester landscape.

Locales as different as the New York Hilton Midtown hotel and the East Hampton Airport (HTOM) are also home to urban honeybees, and thousands those tiny workers have become part of the local landscape.

***

By this point, I had read over two dozen books about honeybees, watched every documentary I could find on Netflix or Social Media, and was rapidly becoming obsessed about anything and everything to do with honeybees. Unfortunately, I could not find many first-person MS BVT testimonials about other people's quests for improved health.

I did learn about a number of Lyme disease recoveries, and read about lots of people whose arthritis had been lessened with the help of bee venom therapy. But when it came to MS, Pat Wagner was the only author with MS that I could find who had shared the story of her illness and recovery. Once again, my amateur status was not helping me connect with or find stories that would continue to inspire and motivate me. There was the doctor who ate nine different vegetables every single day, and was able to exchange her wheelchair for a bicycle. There was the artist in London whose chemist husband helped her defeat her MS with huge strong doses of antibiotics, but when it came to other people fighting MS with BVT, it was hard for me to not feel as if I just might be out there on my own.

While I was discouraged by my inability to find fellow MS bee devotees, there was no way I could deny the fact that both my left arm and hand were stronger, my legs rarely spasmed anymore, the pervasive fog of depression seemed to be slowly lifting, my hair and nails were much-improved, and I could almost feel "the old me" gradually resurfacing.

I had been warned that this process was going to be long and slow, and there was no way I was going to turn my back on any possibility (no matter how remote) of becoming healthy again. I hadn't been able to find a tribe of fellow MS sufferers who were willing to share their stories or get several dozen stings each and every week, but—placebo or not—I was determined to give our Thursday afternoon sting sessions my best shot.

For once, I was willing to quit being impatient, and heed Aesop's wisdom. I relished the opportunity to become the tortoise instead of the hare, and it didn't matter where—city, country, suburbs, etc.—I got my weekly dose of bee venom.

WHAT THE HONEYBEES TAUGHT ME

- According to Guillermo Fernandez, the executive director of New York's Bee Conservatory, "A hive is a box of calm in a frantic city. The buzz and gentleness is quite soothing."
- No matter where (or how) they live, honeybees are almost miraculously adaptive to whatever their environment—rooftop, backyard flower garden, a farmer's field, or orchard—might be.
- Consistently making miniscule baby-step improvements can eventually change—in a positive way—every single aspect of your existence.
- In life, there will always be authority figures (medical or otherwise) who will make pronouncements about what they perceive to be the truth. Sometimes, it can make more sense to listen to what your own internal voice has to say.
- As Roald Dahl (1916-1990) wisely wrote, *"...watch with glittering eyes the whole world around you*

because the greatest secrets are always hidden in the most unlikely of places. Those who don't believe in magic will never find it."

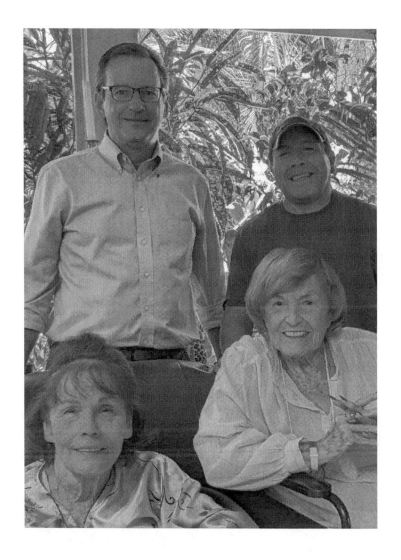

**The Thursday bee sting foursome:
Michael, Ramon, Jeanne, and Marilyn**

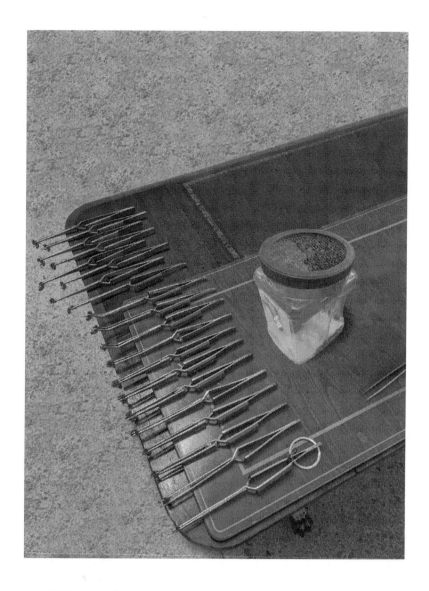

**How the bees arrive at my home,
and how they are prepared for stings.**

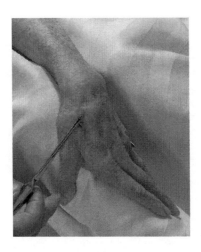

Marilyn's hand getting stung at
the acupuncture "Hegu" point (Li4)

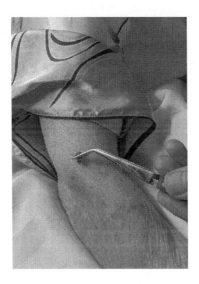

Marilyn's arm getting stung at
the acupuncture "Qu Chi" point (Li11)

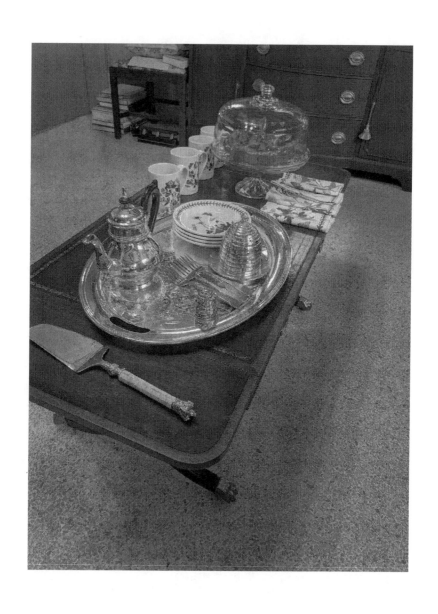

Thursday treat:
Jeanne's strawberry cheesecake

Chapter 9
Celebrity Connections

Not everything that is faced can be changed.
But nothing can be changed until it is faced.
James Baldwin (1924-1987)

The first time I saw my byline in print was when I edited the local summer school newsletter—at age eleven—way back in 1960. Books, the printed word, and reading were important to (and treasured by) our small family. I was lucky enough to have been given a book-centric early childhood that involved my parents reading to me before every afternoon nap and at bedtime until—as a Kindergarten student—my (patient) father taught me how to read. And for more nights than I can tally (long after I was safely tucked into bed) I fell asleep to the distant sound of Mamma and Daddy reading out loud to each other.

As a youngster, in addition to passionately loving the written word, I also developed a life-long sense of no-holds-barred curiosity, which affected every aspect of my life. It extended to what I read as well as (later) to everything I would write. Mentally, I was like an annoying preschooler who never stops asking *"Why?"*

As time went on, that all-consuming curiosity extended (primarily) to the "How?" and "Why?" of other people's lives. In my own life, I still have to be careful to not be invasive or snoopy when it comes to asking people potentially awkward questions about their lives. But the good news is that it's the ideal trait to possess if you're an ambitious author or a foreign journalist who is assigned to write deadline-sensitive celebrity profiles.

One of the most unexpected and enjoyable aspects of my happy and fulfilling career was being able to live a life that could be described as "A-list adjacent." For years, I was able to visit celebrities' homes, attend their parties, ask them probing questions, receive unexpected phone calls from them when they just wanted to chat, share spectacular events together, and enjoy elegant festivities on the fringes of (their) fame.

For someone who grew up in a variety of small West Coast towns, it was a thrill to be the smallest fish in a huge pond overflowing with household-name celebrities. I never took for granted how lucky I was to visit Jane Seymour's homes (both in LA and the UK), be invited to lunch at best-selling author Barbara Taylor Bradford's lavish Mayfair flat, or attend Michael Caine's parties at his Beverly Hills home. I don't mind admitting that I was thrilled to rub shoulders with Anthony Hopkins, Jamie Lee Curtis, and Lifa Vanderpump, or get unexpected phone calls at home from celebrities like Judy Blume, Patrick Duffy, and Audrey Hepburn.

Chronicling the ups and downs of famous musicians, movie stars, or authors could be considered a lightweight assignment for a serious "hard news" journalist, but I have always been hopelessly intrigued by the wide variety of different ways that others choose to navigate through their lives. I loved spending time with Donna Summer's and learning about her strong religious faith, and I was inspired when Gloria Estefan told me about her grueling physical therapy regimen after her 1990 tour bus accident. That sort of voyeuristic curiosity is simply part of my DNA, because I've never stopped wondering what lies beneath the choices and decisions that other people have made.

I had the good fortune to work for a variety of gifted no-nonsense editors who recognized my desire (and determination) to get interesting and useful information out of the celebrities I was assigned to write about. I welcomed every single assignment, whether it was Tim Conway (*The Carol Burnett Show*), Jane Curtin (*Saturday Night Live*), Charles Dance (*Alien* and *Me Before You*), Kirk Douglas (*Spartacus*), Ian McShane (*Lovejoy* and *John Wick*), or Christopher Reeve (*Superman*). And I enjoyed the challenge of turning in copy that contained "insights" that other journalists might have unintentionally overlooked because they were not as compulsively curious as yours truly.

My "need to know" really went into high gear when I was able to interview best-selling authors whose books I had enjoyed. I don't mind confessing that when face-to-face with a talented wordsmith, I often had to remind myself not to feel starstruck or act like a "fan girl." I treasured getting to know gifted writers like Rick Atkinson, A. Scott Berg, Pat Booth, Ray Bradbury, Wayne Dyer, Jane Heller, Ben Stein, Adela Rogers St. Johns, Fay Weldon, and so many others.

***

Once I finally accepted my MS diagnosis, my never-ending curiosity rose to an entirely different level when I began to notice that quite a few celebrities were also embarking on a battle with this challenging illness. In one way, it was mildly comforting to know that I wasn't the only person on the planet forced to cope with such a serious neurological problem. But I also found it sad that other people were being compelled to wrestle with the same often overwhelming difficulties that I had to face day after day.

Many people confuse MS with Muscular Dystrophy, Cerebral Palsy, or a number of other illnesses that can seriously compromise mobility. Essentially, Multiple Sclerosis literally means "many scars," because damaging lesions develop on the white matter of the brain and spinal cord. At its core, MS is a de-myelinating disease that attacks the insulating tissues that surround nerve cells. When the all-important myelin sheath is damaged, the body's nervous system can no longer transmit signals from the brain to the muscles.

Like so many others, when I was diagnosed I didn't know much about MS, but—after a lifetime of being told (and believing) that I was an extraordinarily healthy person—I do remember being terrified at the prospect of dealing with a life-altering, progressive, serious illness.

As I've mentioned before, every case of MS is different, which is one reason why it can take so long to receive a definitive diagnosis. Some of the "tell-tale" symptoms can include balance difficulty, temporary blindness, challenging bathroom issues, dizziness, double vision, fatigue, muscular weakness, mobility problems, numbness, sensitivity to heat, spasticity, and tingling.

The bitter truth is that I have never found it "easy" to live with MS, but when I get exhausted, overheated, catch a cold, or am exposed to any external complicating factor (like the COVID-19 vaccination), the physical challenges I experience increase exponentially. Again, this is probably difficult for an able-bodied person to grasp, but when my body is forced to cope with an additional "stressor", what little muscular strength I still have tends to (literally) evaporate. My one usable extremity—my left arm—becomes so compromised that my fingers lose the ability to push the buttons on the TV remote or on my telephone. During those miserable episodes, which (fortunately) seldom last longer than 24 hours, it feels as if I'm being forced to live inside an iron lung machine.

According to the National Multiple Sclerosis Society, there are currently almost a million people in the US who have been diagnosed with MS. And while most of us struggle with this disease anonymously, there are a growing number of household-name individuals who either have the disease, or have a relative who has been diagnosed. Below is a list of 29 accomplished creative individuals who now have membership in a neurologically-challenged club that no one ever wants to join.

***

- **Art Alexakis**: The *Everclear* singer and songwriter, who has become a political activist on behalf of abuse awareness, drug issues, and military families. Following a car accident, he was diagnosed with MS in 2016, when he was 49 years old.
- **Christina Applegate:** The popular film and TV actress—who became a star on *Married with Children* and *Dead to Me*—announced her diagnosis in 2021, when she was 49 years old. The following year, she received a star on Hollywood's Walk of Fame.
- **Trevor M. Bayne:** Born in 1991, this American stock car racing driver is the youngest person—one day after his 20th birthday—to ever win the Daytona 500. His career began when he started racing go-karts as a five-year-old. He credits his strong faith (and his involvement with Back2Back Ministries) with helping him handle sudden fame, as well as his 2013 MS diagnosis when he was only 22. At first, he experienced blurred vision, fatigue, nausea, and numbness, but he is currently symptom free.
- **Selma Blair:** The movie and TV actress revealed her diagnosis in 2018, and three years later she released a documentary (*Introducing Selma Blair*) about her arduous MS journey. In 2022, when she was 50, she published her best-selling memoir *Mean Baby*, and appeared on *Dancing with the Stars*.

- **Bryan Bickell:** This Canadian former professional Ice Hockey star was a member of the Stanley Cup-winning Chicago Black Hawks when, starting in 2015, his symptoms of leg and shoulder pain forced him to miss multiple games. In 2016, when he was 30 years old, he was diagnosed with MS; Bickel retired the following year.
- **Neil Cavuto**: The Fox News Anchor and business journalist hosts three different TV programs. In 1997, when he was 39 years old, after he'd survived a cancer battle, Cavuto learned that he had MS. He is the author of two New York Times best-selling books.
- **Benjamin J. Cohen**: This British LGBTQ and disability rights campaigner is the CEO of *PinkNews*, as well as a contributor to the London *Evening Standard News Paper*. Diagnosed with MS after joining Channel 4 News in 2006, when he was only 23 years old, he now serves on the board of trustees of the UK branch of Handicap International.
- **Richard M. Cohen:** This three-time Emmy-award winning journalist and author has worked for both CBS and CNN. The husband of Meredith Vieira, he was diagnosed in 1973, when he was 25 years old.
- **Jason DaSilva**: In 2005, Emmy-winning documentary filmmaker DaSilva began having trouble with his vision as well as with his ability to walk. Soon afterwards, he was diagnosed with primary progressive multiple sclerosis (PPMS). His landmark films (*When I Walk* and *When We Walk*) are designed to chronicle his journey with MS. He is the founder of AXS Map, which helps those of us who

are disabled find accessible public spaces, restaurants, restrooms, and stores.

- **Janice Dean**: In 2005, when she was 35, Dean—a Canadian-born American meteorologist on *FOX & Friends*—was diagnosed with MS. She has written a series of children's books, as well as two memoirs.
- **Joan Didion** (1934-2021): After experiencing bouts of partial blindness in 1972, when she was 38 years old, the celebrated author was diagnosed with MS. Luckily, the disease remained in remission for the rest of her life. She wrote about her diagnosis in her best-selling non-fiction book *Slouching Toward Bethlehem.*
- **Rita Dove**: The first African-American Poet Laureate (and prolific author) was diagnosed with MS in 1997, when she was 45 years old. She publicly acknowledged having MS for the first time in her latest book, *Playlist for the Apocalypse: Poems.* Born in 1952, Dove has admitted that she is no longer able to write her poems by hand.
- **Annette Funicello** (1942-2013): The popular singer, TV, and movie actress, who began her career as a member of the original *Mickey Mouse Club,* revealed her diagnosis in 1987. She was the first household-name celebrity to "go public" with her MS disability.
- **Barbara Jordan (1936-1996):** This Civil Rights activist was the first African-American Texas state senator, and, in 1973 she was the first Southern African-American woman elected to the state's house of Representatives. Her MS symptoms began surfacing in 1973, her 1976 speech at the Democratic National Convention keynote address has been listed

as number five in American Rhetoric's top 100 speeches of the 20th century. In 1994, President Clinton awarded her the Presidential Medal of Freedom.

- **Jonathan Katz**: This Emmy-winning actor, comedian, and voice actor, whose parents immigrated from Hungary, was diagnosed in 1996, when he was 49 years old. He has since become a spokesperson for an MS medication manufacturer.
- **John Michael Kosterlitz**: Is a British-American physicist who has been a professor at Brown University since 1982. He was diagnosed in 1973, when he was 35 years old, and in 2016 he won the Nobel prize in physics.
- **John King**: CNN's chief national correspondent is also the host of *Inside Politics*. In 2021, he revealed that he had been diagnosed with MS back in 2008 (when he was 45), but had kept the news secret from both colleagues as well as friends. He chose to go public about having MS because he wanted to speak out about the importance of COVID-19 vaccines and mask mandates to help the immunocompromised individuals.
- **Jack Osbourne**: After battling depression and substance abuse issues, the son of heavy-metal singer Ozzy Osbourne and Sharon Osbourne is a popular English media personality. At age 27, in 2012, he was diagnosed with MS, and since then, he has become an advocate for MS research and healthy lifestyle choices.
- **Alan and David Osmond**: Part of the legendary Osmonds music group, which often performed on

CBS in the 1960s, Alan Osmond was diagnosed with MS in 1987 when he was 38 years old. His son, David, was also diagnosed in 2005 when he was 26 years old. The recipient of the Dorothy Corwin Spirit of Life Award from the National Multiple Sclerosis Society, Alan's motto is: "I may have MS, but MS does NOT have me!"

- **Jacqueline du Pré** (1945-1987): One of the greatest celloists of all time, this British musician began her professional career at Wigmore Hall in London when she was only 16 years old. Eleven years later, her 1973 MS diagnosis derailed her brilliant career when she was only 27 years old.

- **Richard Pryor** (1940-2005): The popular groundbreaking comedian—who had struggled with drug addiction issues—was diagnosed in 1986, when he was 46 years old.

- **Frasier C. Robinson III** (1935-1991): Michelle Obama's father was diagnosed in 1967, while in his early 30s. In her memoir (*Becoming*), she wrote poignantly about how painful it was to watch him go to work every day when simply being able to stand or walk involved so much effort.

- **Anne Rowling (1945-1990):** J.K. Rowling's (*Harry Potter*) mother was finally diagnosed in 1980 (when she was 35), after developing a variety of unpleasant symptoms over several years. Her illness surprised the family because she had been physically fit, and neither drank nor smoked. The author began writing the first *Harry Potter* book six months before her mother died in 1990.

- **Ann Romney**: Perhaps best known as the wife of Massachusetts Governor, Utah Senator, and presidential candidate Mitt Romney, she has been a powerful health advocate. Diagnosed with MS in 1998, when she was 49 years old, she has combined mainstream and alternative treatments to help diminish her symptoms. In 2014 she opened the Ann Romney Center for Neurological Diseases at Brigham and Women's Hospital in Boston.
- **Gordon Schumer**: In 1993, when comedian Amy Schumer was only twelve years old, her father was diagnosed with MS. In her memoir (*The Girl with the Lower Back Tattoo*) and her hit movie (*Trainwreck*), she reveals the devastation his illness had on their family. She has raised hundreds of thousands of dollars on behalf of the National Multiple Sclerosis Society.
- **Jamie Lynn Sigler**: Although she had been diagnosed in 2001, with the help her colleagues, the *Sopranos* actress did not reveal that she had MS until 2016. Currently, she is a reoccurring cast member of ABC's *Big Sky*.
- **Clay Walker**: This platinum award-winning country singer songwriter was 26 years old when he was diagnosed in 1996. In 2003, he established a non-profit charity (*Band Against MS*), and has been awarded a Humanitarian Award for his fundraising efforts, which include a charity golf tournament.
- **Montel Williams**: The popular Marine Corps veteran and talk show host was diagnosed in 1999, when he was 33. He has switched from the use of traditional

pharmaceuticals to alternative treatments, including the use of Cannabis.

- **Walter Williams:** This Rock and Roll Hall of Fame O'Jays (*Love Train*) singer was diagnosed in 1983, just before his 40th birthday. His symptoms began with numbness in his toes, which soon spread from his foot all the way up his leg; at one point, he felt completely numb from the waist down. After a month of feeling depressed and frightened, he began a strict regimen of exercising, watching his diet, and becoming proactive regarding his MS. Williams is now a paid spokesman for Biogen IDEC, the biotech company that makes AVONEX, which he takes to treat his relapsing, remitting form of this disease.

WHAT THE HONEYBEES TAUGHT ME

- Illness can visit anyone, regardless of accomplishment, age, fame, talent, virtue or wealth. Sadly, whether you are a honeybee or a human being, life can sometimes be both perilous and unpredictable.
- Medical experts insist that MS patients' symptoms cannot improve, and can only be "managed" with costly chemical medications. But it's a safe bet that *Apis mellifera* worker bees would disagree, as do I…
- MS patients are usually warned that although their lifespan will be shortened, the disease won't kill them. Perhaps the hardworking honeybee instinctively know that they too have a limited time to live, which is why they make the most of every single moment.

- When it comes to illness, injury, or random misfortune, honeybees know only too well that their fellow hive inhabitants will never offer support or sympathy. The lesson for the rest of us may be to simply—no matter what—quit whining to others whenever life's burdens seem overwhelming. Just like the bees, no one likes complainer.
- Worker bees understand that—whatever their ability, e.g., making Royal Jelly, creating beeswax, etc.— they can only do that specific job temporarily. As we "lose" various abilities due to accident, age, illness, disease, or misuse, it can help to remember that nothing we are ever able to accomplish or do comes with a "Lifetime Warranty." Awareness of MS has increased to the point where even popular network TV shows (like *West Wing's* President Josiah Bartlett and *The Resident's* Dr. Randolph Bell) share with audiences the diverse challenges of this enigmatic neurological progressive illness.

Chapter 10
The Queen

Heavy is the head that wears the crown.
HENRY THE IV, PART II
Shakespeare (1564-1616)

Up to this point, I've been very comfortable about accepting and acknowledging my status as an enthusiastic well-read (but untrained) amateur when it comes to the mysterious world of honeybees. A part of me will always be a bit self-conscious about admiring honeybees so much, yet having far too little technical knowledge, hands-on experience, or academic background regarding their lives to ever be considered an "expert."

When I consulted the *Oxford English Dictionary* about the various levels aspects of expertise, however, I found a way to diminish my self-doubt. According to the OED, an expert is *"A person with special knowledge, skill, or training in something."* And after several years of close to 50 in-person bee stings each and every week—plus hundreds of hours devoted to bee magazines, books, conversations, documentaries and on-line sites—I've definitely compiled plenty of "special" due-diligence research.

Conventional wisdom would like us to believe that the hive is populated by pre-programmed worker bees who slavishly devote their lives to the care and feeding of the hive's only fertile female. In fact, the worker bees need and respond to the *Apis mellifera* Queen Bee's various pheromone levels because they provide essential feedback about her physical well-being, which is essential to the health and survival of the hive.

Without a Queen Bee, a cell or colony or hive simply cannot exist. Fortunately, every hatched larvae that becomes a worker bee seems to be born with the knowledge that keeping the Queen alive and well is absolutely essential to their own (as well as everyone else's) lifespan. Oddly enough, a Queen Bee (who can live for up to six years) hatches after only 16 days, while a worker bee (which only lives for six weeks) needs 21 days. The Queen's shorter gestation period, is puzzling in light of the fact that—unlike a worker bee—her body is considerably larger, and she has a fully-functioning reproductive system.

As far as I could tell, only two things made a difference between a developing *Apis mellifera* Queen Bee and a developing worker bee. One difference is that they grow in different-sized spaces, eggs will look like commas in their brood cells. The Queen will lay different sorts of eggs in different spots in the honeycomb. A larger drone cell will get an unfertilized egg, which will become a male bee. A regular-sized cell gets a fertilized egg, which (most of the time) will become a worker.

The other distinguishing feature is that they receive different nutrients while developing. After receiving Royal Jelly for the first three days, a worker is then fed a combination of pollen and honey that the nursery bees use to create a type of "beebread." The developing Queens, however, **only** receive Royal Jelly for their entire lives.

I am in awe of all the beekeepers I've met—in person, in the pages of books and magazines, or on the documentaries and TV programs that I've watched. Each seems to possess an exceptional affinity for (and understanding of) the multifaceted world that these mighty little insects have built.

***

A number of my friends—who find my late-life passion for *Apis mellifera* a bit over-the-top and (frankly) puzzling—have jokingly nicknamed me The Queen Bee. And no matter how many times I deflect their teasing and remind them that I'm far from being a true authority, they readily acknowledge that even though I don't sell honey or harvest honeycomb, when it comes to the bees, I'm no longer a novice.

There was a brief moment when I began to convince myself that I was almost ready to shift from "beginner" status to "advanced" standing, but that fleeting wave of self-deception didn't last very long. My good friend, Donna, sent me an amazing (and quite beautiful) hardbound book by Hilary Kearney, a young beekeeper in San Diego, and the founder of "Girl Next Door Honey." Her book (*QueenSpotting: Meet the Remarkable Queen Bee and Discover the Drama at the Heart of the Hive*) taught me—in no uncertain terms—that I will probably never acquire the bee-centric skills to advance from simply being a knowledgeable bee aficionado to a bona-fide *Apis mellifera* expert.

In San Diego, Kearney manages 90 hives, writes about bees for *The Huffington Post, Mother Earth News,* as well as *Vogue,* and has become the enthusiastic face of urban beekeeping in Southern California. I read her 127-page book in one sitting but failed miserably when I arrived at her challenge to "spot the Queen." The artwork in Kearney's book includes 48 beautiful up-close color photographs that capture hundreds of worker bees while they go about their essential duties, and care for the Queen. The book's visual "task" is for the reader to correctly identify the Queen Bee in each colorful photo.

Sadly, when faced with this stunning honeybee version of *Where's Waldo?,* I simply could not pass the test. All I could see were countless worker bees who were all facing different directions and involved with different tasks. My unqualified and untrained eyes simply could not accurately distinguish between a drone, a worker bee, and—no matter how hard I tried—the Queen.

***

When a hive's worker bees sense (through those all-powerful pheromones) that the Queen Bee is in declining health, and is therefore laying fewer eggs, they begin to construct the groundwork for the creation of a new Queen Bee. This process is called *supersedure,* and begins with the construction of between ten and 20 unique wax "Queen cups" that they build and place around the edges of the existing honeycomb. The Queen then deposits an egg in each one, and over the next two weeks those special cups will grow and become large Queen cells. They actually resemble an unshelled peanut that is hanging from the outer edge of the honeycomb to accommodate the growing larvae. In about fourteen days, the end of the Queen Cup starts to become thin; its papery texture allows the newly-emerging Queen to chew her way out, and begin her new way of life.

If the Queen cups had been built because an overcrowded colony is getting ready to swarm, the new Queens will often not hatch until the existing Queen and her followers (usually about half the hive) have left. But if the cups were built because the existing Queen was ill, there will be a "hostile takeover." In this scenario, there will be a "death by stinging" event as the existing Queen will try to kill her newly "hatched" potential replacement. Following the brutal and dispassionate world of the honeybee hive, it can feel like a real-life Darwinian "survival of the fittest" situation.

If the hive needs a new Queen, they sometimes eliminate the old one by a process called "balling." This is when a small cluster of worker bees crowd around the doomed old Queen and push closer and closer until she is either overheated or squeezed to death. Some beekeepers report that the worker bees are so intent on killing the no-longer viable Queen that they even bite or pull at her legs or wings during the process.

Usually, the first "new" Queen Bee that hatches will then sting any other rivals through the walls of their unopened Queen cups. But, if another potential Queen has already hatched, then the two will face each other and fight till the death. When the Queens fight with each other, they make a special sound—called "piping"—that some beekeepers report resembles the sound of a flute or a duck quacking. This sound is made by the muscles of their four wings, and it signifies the start of a lethal battle. While worker bees are only able to sting once, Queen Bees have a stinger that does not have barbs on it. This means she can sting repeatedly, or—if she chooses—bite or even tear at her opponent's body until she dies.

Worker bees do not use their stinger on the soon-to-be sacrificed Queen. Instead, they might starve her to death, crush her body, or even make sure that she is overheated. The Queen, on the other hand, will only sting other Queens who present a threat to her dominance.

Additionally, a Queen Bee's venom sack is three times the size of a worker bee's. Why? Because during her six-year lifespan, she may need to defend her status numerous times. On the other hand, a defeated Queen will die after about ten or 15 minutes, and the hive's undertaker bees then quickly drag her lifeless body away.

**

Back in the 1980s, the Feminist Movement had just begun to take hold, and usually only one or two "token" women could be found at Board Meetings or in positions of potential power. Remember the achingly realistic movie *Working Girl* or *The Devil Wears Prada?* The executive Females who chose to cling to their own elevated status rather than share their good fortune with other women were derisively referred to as "Queen Bees." During that era, it was definitely not a complimentary term. As a working woman, I had met a few of them, and vowed to never behave the way they did.

As I learned more and more about the *Apis mellifera* Queen Bee, I began to realize that a not-so-distant part of me could actually relate to parts of her unusual lifestyle. The Queen Bee is totally dependent on other females to prop her up and support her during every single day of her life. Because she usually only leaves the hive—after her 16-day gestation period—for her "Nuptial Flight," she essentially spends the bulk of her life in the dark, surrounded by a rotating cast of several thousand worker bees who care for her. They feed the Queen, groom her, make sure she is hydrated, and provide housing for the thousands of eggs she lays each day. She is literally dependent on the kindness of others. Playwright Tennessee Williams (1911–1983) would classify her as an insect version of Blanche duBois from his play *Cat On A Hot Tin Roof.*

Throughout her six-year lifespan, as many as eight different generations of workers will keep her environment clean and comfortable, and make sure that she has everything she could possibly need or want. Bees who live where the weather gets cold in the wintertime have a unique way of protecting their Queen. In icy weather, they create a softball-sized cluster around her to keep the temperature close to 95 degrees, and as the mercury rises the size of the *Apis mellifera* insulation gets larger and larger until their group heat machine is no longer needed.

Essentially, worker bees know that they must do everything possible to protect their "mother" from any and all irritants or dangers. To make sure that absolutely nothing at all ever interferes with their Queen's vital egg-laying duties, they even remove her excrement!

Whether it's through instinct or pheromones (or both), the little worker honeybees seem to live in a never-ending cycle of compulsory cooperation that lets them know exactly how to keep their Queen (as well as their hive) on track.

***

In the long-ago days when I had an executive position in the media world, and was often the only female in the room, I did my best to help ambitious and talented women enjoy the few professional perks that had come my way. I made a concentrated effort to NOT be a 1980s Queen Bee. Several decades later, however, as a profoundly disabled, unemployable, seriously-handicapped, and heartbroken recent widow, I discovered that without the kind hearts and caring acts of my many girlfriends, I would have been—much like an ill *Apis mellifera* Queen Bee—well and truly doomed.

In 2017, every single aspect of my once-seemingly pleasant life was under threat. Emotionally, financially, and physically I felt too weary and far too frightened to survive the nightmarish scenario that I was being forced to face. In the past, as a younger woman, I had always been strong enough to—one way or another—eventually overcome whatever difficulties happened to come my way. But after the death of my supportive (often uxorious) husband, and the unwelcome arrival of what seemed like an insurmountable dump truck full of continual real-world adversity, I was ready to give up. There was simply no strength left in me to even think about pretending to be positive or strong. My Stubborn Optimism had taken a lengthy and unscheduled sabbatical. And, of course, the worst thing in the world for someone with MS is continual stress...

That grim time was when a devoted army of my friends—some from high school, some from college, some from Los Angeles, some from London, some from Florida—essentially took over my life. Like the energetic workers in a honeybee hive, my tribe of true-blue friends each graciously managed to reach out to let me know that they were sure (and would personally see to it) that my tsunami of troubles would only be temporary.

Now, when I look back on those deeply sad and scary days, all I remember is that until they stepped in, I felt as if I had simply run out of fuel; the prospect of having to face yet another painful day filled me with dread. I have no clear memory of exactly who did what (and when) during those dark days, but I knew that a great deal of (very) heavy lifting was involved. Some friends brought meals, some wrote checks and paid bills, some drove me to my doctor appointments, some took me to meetings with attorneys and bankers, while others regularly stayed with me at night to make sure I wasn't sitting alone in the dark and crying.

Their coordinated group effort helped me to (eventually) dry my tears, and quit feeling sorry for myself. One clever friend created and managed a GoFundMe account, which helped me save my home, and several others took turns flying long distances to be with me, to dilute my sorrow, and lessen my loneliness. Another angel unearthed my address and phone lists, and contacted people she'd never met before in order to make sure that even more friends who knew or cared about me fully understood that I was in a dangerous world of hurt, and needed all the help that could be assembled.

For months, I was lucky enough to live in my own private and very protected Queen cell because I was surrounded by a Heaven-sent hive of concerned friends who made it their mission to care for and protect me for as long as necessary.

**

The honeybee Queen, which does not have a pollen pouch (officially known as *corbiculae*) has a long and elegantly tapered body that is almost twice the length of a worker. Some observers swear that her legs are so delicate they resemble a spider's. And because of her daily egg-laying duties—she deposits an egg in a honeycomb cell about every 30 seconds—her abdomen looks both heavy and large. A Queen will sometimes begin laying her eggs in the middle of the honeycomb and then continue the process in concentric circles. But spatial preferences aside, for the majority of her life, a Queen will be surrounded by devoted much-younger workers who keep their antenna, their eyes, and sometimes even their front legs (where arms would be) as close as possible to their Queen's body.

Every Queen Bee has her own unique pheromones. This is important because when the workers are old enough (and their wings are strong enough) to hunt for nectar and pollen, they use their knowledge of her unique smell to guide them safely back to their hive.

The new Queen emerges from her large cell after about two weeks of development, and she remains inside the hive for another three to seven days before she takes her all-important Nuptial Flight. This can take anywhere from five minutes to half an hour, and a number of different male drones are usually involved. The Nuptial Flight usually takes place only a few miles away from the hive, and over fifty feet high in the air. Perhaps this is to ensure that only the strongest drones will pass their DNA to future worker bee generations. Sometimes there are as many as a dozen different matings, and the result will be enough sperm to fertilize hundreds of thousands of eggs. After her Nuptial (or Maiden) flight the Queen returns to the hive with over five million sperm stored inside her, and within only a few days her life-long egg laying career will officially begin. When the Queen lays an egg, it resembles a tiny vertically-placed grain of rice that has been placed inside a honeycomb cell.

If—for any reason—the Queen is unable to leave the hive for a Nuptial Flight (for example, due to bad weather) she will remain infertile and be labeled a "drone layer." This means she is unable to produce female worker bees, and this discovery will result in the other hive members killing her; a Queen that cannot produce worker bees puts the entire hive at peril.

Sometimes, when a new Queen has been imported into a hive she will announce her presence with a sound that has been compared with a kazoo or a teakettle's whistle. It is a staccato high-pitched sound that lets her new subjects know that their new Queen has arrived, and that regulated and ordinary honeybee life can soon resume.

The amount of eggs that a Queen lays each day can be greater than her own body weight. The Queen controls the hive through a variety of pheromones, each of which serves a specific purpose. One of them actually prevents the development of ovaries in the worker bees, which makes it impossible for them to lay viable eggs.

The Queen is the only bee in the hive whose wings do not touch the end of her abdomen. This is because that area of her body is designed to be large enough to contain a lifetime's worth of eggs and sperm. While worker bees and drones have furry backs, the Queen's is shiny; also, many Queens have light-colored legs, while the drones and worker bees have dark ones. The Queen's legs are longer and thinner than the ones of the other hive's inhabitants because she does not have the pollen sacks on them that the other worker bees do.

***

Years ago, long before I began my bee sting experiment, a dear friend from California arrived for a short visit. She'd known me when I had been so fit and young that we'd all believed I would always enjoy an independent, productive, and self-sufficient lifestyle. My caring friend watched the way my much-cherished and essential Guatemalan caregiver, Ramon, and I navigated our way through each day's challenges. Concerned about my paralysis, she asked, *"From the time you wake up until lights out, how many times do you say **Gracias**, **Por Favor**, and **Thank You** each and every day?"*

I admitted that I'd never bothered to keep track, but it was—sadly—probably well over a hundred. Because I only had the use of my left arm, my caring friend soon realized that there was no way for me to survive without continual help on a daily basis. As much as I hated to admit it, my MS muscle failure had made it practically impossible for me to do much of anything without asking for another person's assistance.

That visit took place over four years ago, and after I'd had about 100 sessions with Michael, I noticed a curious (and very encouraging) development. One evening in early 2022, it dawned on me that I was asking for help—from Ramon, from girlfriends, from visitors—far less often than I had previously done. Without any excitement or fanfare, I realized that my body was slowly and gradually changing. My left hand could grasp better. My left arm could stretch farther. My hand-eye coordination had definitely improved, and—for the first time in years—I could pick things up off the floor by myself, and even drink from a glass without using a straw.

I decided to ask Ramon, who (for close to two decades) has spent hours each day by my side, if he had noticed a positive physiological change as well. After he nodded enthusiastically, I then asked him how many times each day—of late—I usually asked him for help. He gave the matter some thought, and then smiled before answering "*Menos de quarenta* (Fewer than 40)."

Of course, I still needed help to put on and take off clothes and shoes, get groomed, move from any point A to any point B, and to get food and water (or better yet, chocolate and coffee). But there was no doubt that without any pharmaceutical involvement whatsoever my balance, hair, nails, skin, and strength had all **begun to improve**. Even though such good news was against all odds (and in spite of what the different doom-and-gloom doctors had told me on a daily basis) I had far fewer muscle spasms, and a whole lot less pain.

The bottom line was that it was getting a lot easier for me to simply live my MS-altered life. There will, of course, always be skeptics, as well as individuals who question the ability of our bodies to heal without employing prescribed medication. All I can say is that for the first time in years I could see enough measurable improvement to experience the best feeling of all: **HOPE**.

WHAT THE HONEYBEES TAUGHT ME

- Back in 1919, the English author Daisy Ashford (1881-1972) wrote *The Young Visitors,* and correctly observed that *Being royal has many painful drawbacks.*
- Attention to detail, helping hands, and small acts of kindness can sustain (as well as transform) a life. This applies to human beings as well as to honeybees.
- Not everyone can do everything, but everyone can do something.
- Sometimes, even those of us who are (or like to think of ourselves as) independent, powerful or strong, need to (kindly) be cared for helped.
- Watching the honeybees' inherent lack of empathy, and the transactional tendencies of the hive culture, helped me appreciate and treasure my friends' astonishing altruism even more than I already did.

Chapter 11
Traveling Honeybees

Change in all things is sweet.
Aristotle (384-322 BCE)

There have been many external forces that converged to make me the woman I am today, and one of the most influential occurred when I was 16 years old. That's when I passed my DMV driver's test, and had the wherewithal to savor the sensation (within the limits of a small California town) of traveling when and where I wanted to.

Two years later, I used the money that I'd earned (from babysitting and ironing for frazzled housewives or filing documents in my father's First American Title Company office) to purchase my very first car. For $500, I acquired a 1960 red Austin-Healey Sprite with a wounded transmission that was missing a tooth out of first gear. My father could see how much I loved that little sports car, so he taught me how to drive a stick shift, and how to start my snazzy little red car in second gear. And that's how and when my life-long love affair with travel began in earnest...

Since that time, I've been lucky enough to own a variety of enviable (mostly foreign) automobiles, but all that changed when—in the late 1990s—my progressive disability status made it impossible to continue driving the blue hand-controlled Oldsmobile sedan that ultimately became my last car. (FYI: The key to driving when my legs no longer worked, was to rely on hand-controls that were attached to the steering column. I pressed down on the left lever to accelerate, and pressed inwards on the right lever to brake. It's an easy skill to master, and one that allows people with disabilities to once again feel mobile, as well as part of the world at large.) These days, since my right arm continues to ignore the signals that my brain tries to send it, my wheelchair and I travel around town in a handicap-accessible Dodge van, where I am a passenger, and someone else controls the steering wheel.

Before MS altered everything in my life, I was one of those lucky people who leapt at the chance to visit new places. My passport was always in my purse, I had no fear of flying whatsoever, and I wholeheartedly embraced the concept of change as well as the thrill of travel. Now, however, I barely recognize the woman I've become, who is actively change-resistant, and suffers from a decades-long case of terminal cabin fever. A huge part of my psyche wishes that—like the honeybees—I could always be in constant motion.

***

I'm embarrassed to admit that before I became *Apis mellifera*-obsessed, I had no idea that every year millions of honeybees are transported on giant 18-wheeler trucks all across the United States to serve as "mobile pollinators" for America's agricultural industry. In the first study conducted in 20 years for

167

the Florida State Beekeepers Association by the Food and Resource Economics Department of the University of Florida's Institute of Food and Agricultural Services, my state alone generates over $30 million in long-distance crop pollination services.

Obviously, transporting large numbers of bees only really became possible when the automobile industry was in its infancy during the early 1900s. Before that time, when beekeepers tried to move hives using horse-drawn wagons, when the bees got angry, their equine-directed stings would make the process both challenging and costly. Plus, if beekeepers tried to use railroad travel to move their honeybees, there was no way to ensure that the bees would be properly cared for during transport.

Moving the honeybees by placing them on trucks took a grand step forward when both the Bobcat forklift (which has the ability to make sharp turns) and the introduction of sturdy wood pallets made it possible to move half a dozen hives at a time onto trucks. These developments eliminated horses getting attacked by angry *Apis mellifera*, as well as train delays and water shortages killing honeybees on railroad cars.

If you happen to see—while driving (particularly at night when its cooler) on I-95 or Route 66 or Highway 30—a large flat-bed truck loaded with hundreds of square white boxes covered with netting, you are probably catching a glimpse of a commercial beekeeper enterprise. Those giant trucks are headed to an agricultural destination for a particular crop that needs to be pollinated. Approximately two thirds of the 2.9 million honeybee hives in the country spend at least some of their short lifetime travelling from one state to another. The five-ton trucks are usually about 35 feet long, eight feet wide, twelve feet high, and loaded with over 450 active beehives. That translates into a "load" of about 26 million honeybees.

When the truck drivers reach each of their designated stops during their pilgrimage, the hungry *Apis mellifera* will gorge themselves on one specific type of nectar until their hives are reloaded on the 18 wheelers, and then they are driven to the next crop that needs to be pollinated. The list of America's farm products that are honeybee dependent includes everything from almonds, apples, blueberries, broccoli, cranberries, cucumbers, melons, onions, pumpkins, raspberries, squash, as well as others.

In today's America, about $15 billion worth of agricultural crops are pollinated each year, and honeybees are responsible for at least 80% of the total work involved. No one knows exactly why *Apis mellifera* pollination seems to create a bigger harvest and better quality of a variety of produce—whether its berries, fruits, seeds, or vegetables. But we do know that in 2012, the USDA did a study that showed orchards that had a healthy honeybee population enjoyed a 25 percent increase in fruit production.

Commercial beekeepers who transport their honeybees from one crop to another must concentrate their efforts on running the business of moving the bees that pollinate crops and making a profit while doing so. Here is a brief glimpse into the working world of migratory honeybees, and a tiny hint of the huge impact they have on America's agricultural well-being:

ALABAMA has a small but significant (about 160,000 acres) annual harvest of soybeans that need to be pollinated, and triple that amount of land occupied by cotton fields. These two important crops depend directly on honeybee pollination for both the quality and quantity of their harvests.

During the time when my family lived in Yuma, **ARIZONA**, the three crops I remembered seeing most often were cantaloupe, cotton, and sugar beets. Today, melons are considered to be an $80 million crop, and honeybee pollination increases their sweetness, volume, and weight. To give you an idea of how long ago my Arizona residency was, in those days we could stop at any one of dozens of roadside stands and purchase thirteen (called a "baker's dozen") large freshly-picked cantaloupes for a single dollar bill. Today, at my local Trader Joe's market, just one (rather small) melon was priced at $3.99.

ARIZONA, **FLORIDA**, **GEORGIA**, and **TEXAS** produce close to four billion pounds of watermelon each year, and since its pollen is sticky. *Apis mellifera* is needed to successfully pollinate each plant. Honeybees need to visit a watermelon flower close to eight times in order to create a large, perfectly-shaped fruit. The plant's flowers open first thing in the morning and then close by early afternoon, so the honeybees need to visit the plants as early as possible each day.

CALIFORNIA is responsible for about 80% of the almonds grown worldwide. This crop alone covers close to 800,000 acres of land, and it takes about a million colonies (hives) of honeybees to successfully pollinate such an essential harvest. While most other crops only need to have one hive per acre, for adequate pollination almond trees require two.

Since almond trees seem to have a three-decade viable productive lifespan, farmers have begun planting almond orchards in a diamond pattern using two additional rows of trees, which has altered the existing pollination pattern. For every 130 trees, two or three hives are needed, and this layout makes it easier for beekeepers to place their hives (both in and out) of the orchards.

Almonds are America's seventh most valuable crop, estimated at $6 billion, and they are considered to be the largest pollination-dependent agricultural product grown in America.

Additionally, 90% of domestically grown kiwis also come from California. It's close to a $40 million crop, and the annual output is about 30,000 tons of this increasingly popular nutrient-rich fruit. Just as with several other crops, both male and female flowers are involved in the pollination process.

According to the National Agricultural Statistics Service, 90% of US avocados rely on honeybee pollination even though this is considered a partially self-pollinating crop. And, over 90% of domestic avocados are grown in Southern California.

Before our move to London, whenever I used to drive from Los Angeles to Ventura or Santa Barbara, I would pass by endless acres of strawberry fields, so it didn't surprise me to learn that California is also the world's largest producer of this popular berry. It's a $3 billion crop, and more than three billion pounds of strawberries are grown every year. When pollinated by honeybees, domestic strawberries tend to have a stronger color, fewer deformities, and their firmer skin extends shelf life by more than twelve hours compared with "wind-pollinated" plants.

I have lived in South **FLORIDA** for over 30 years, but I never knew that nearly a quarter of America's 2.6 million bee colonies (600,000) are located in the state where I live, and over 80% of these colonies are owned by commercial beekeepers. Florida happens to be the largest cucumber producing state in America, but until I became honeybee obsessed, I never knew that cucumber plants—like strawberries— have both male and female flowers. The pollen for this fruit is particularly sticky, and it has to be transferred between the two in order to create a fully-formed cucumber. The more times a honeybee visits a cucumber flower, the larger and more attractive the cucumber will be. An open cucumber vine—when properly pollinated—can produce about six fruit per foot.

MICHIGAN is the leading state for growing cherries, which only has a short one-week blossoming period for honeybee pollination. This crop is valued at close to $800 million, and thanks to the traveling honeybees that pollinate about 90% of American cherries, the annual production of this fruit is close to 400,000 tons. Also, the majority of blueberries (which are estimated to be a $600 million crop) are also grown in southwest Michigan. These plants provide both nectar and pollen, and honeybees are responsible for 95% of the essential pollination process.

ILLINOIS, **OHIO**, and **PENNSYLVANIA** produce most of the American gourd, pumpkin, and squash crops; like cucumber, kiwi and strawberry plants, they have both male and female flowers. Again, when pollinated by honeybees the number and the weight of these crops increase. It's estimated that gourds, pumpkin, and squash are a $250 million crop each year.

OREGON is the nation's largest producer of raspberries, which have become close to a $200 million crop. Unlike so many other types of produce, however, raspberries can partially self-fertilize. But with honeybee pollination, the plants are able to produce more fruit and larger berries. Bees are particularly fond of raspberry plants because of their large amount of nectar.

The US is the second largest apple producer in the world, and 25% of all domestically-grown apples are exported. **WASHINGTON** state produces about 70% of our domestic apple crop, closely followed by **NEW YORK**. This $2.7 billion harvest is dependent on honeybees to spread the pollen from one apple tree onto the flowers of another. If there were no bees, the fragrant apple blossoms would still appear, but they would then die without ever creating an edible fruit.

***

The business of moving honeybee hives from one state and one crop to another is worth well over $300 million each year, and the largest number of colonies that move into **CALIFORNIA** (about 60%) each January come from the Northern Great Plains (**MINNESOTA, MONTANA, NORTH DAKOTA,** and **SOUTH DAKOTA**). Honeybees from Western states and the Pacific Northwest account for about 10% each of the total of traveling honeybees that are destined to visit California. When everything works the way it should, the honeybees that travel along America's seasonal agricultural routes contribute three extremely important services: (1) they provide over $300 million worth of pollination for fruits, nuts, seeds, and vegetables, (2) they gather enough forage to produce over $300 million worth of high-quality honey, and (3) while accomplishing the first two feats, some of them can actually help their own colonies thrive and grow stronger.

According to Professor Stashenko, every state in America has at least one crop that relies on "migratory" honeybees for pollination, but it's not, however, all fun and games for those little hard-working honeybees.

Traveling on 18-wheeler flatbed trucks at night from one state to another can result in measurable physical stress and occasional colony loss.

Additionally, if the honeybees are not able to forage adequately while they're being moved, this will result in limited future food for the colony. Frequently, pollinating a single crop may not provide an adequate amount of nutritious high-quality nectar or pollen. Just like humans, honeybees need both carbohydrates (nectar) and proteins (pollen), which is why some beekeepers provide sugar water and "pollen patties" for their tiny workers. Also, the stresses involved with travel-related temperature extremes—either too hot or too cold—is always a serious risk factor.

One sad "traveling honeybee" story happened in early 2022, and it highlighted the potential dangers of transporting live pollinators from one location to another. An Alaskan businesswoman, Sarah McElrea, has a small business that imports *Apis mellifera* for local beekeepers, and helps provide pollination services for apple farmers and nurseries in her state. For years, her standard way of importing the honeybees was to fly them in large crates from Sacramento, California to Seattle, Washington, and then to Anchorage, Alaska. From there, she would distribute the bees to her agricultural clients.

Unfortunately, there was an airplane mix-up, and Delta Airlines mistakenly scheduled the large crates of live pollinating honeybees to be flown to their hub in Atlanta, Georgia, where they were parked on the tarmac. By the time the transport error could be resolved, it was too late for the colonies; as a result of that "mix-up," over six million honeybees perished in the heat.

This is a tragic example of what can go wrong if no one pays close attention to the honeybees' well-being while they are being moved. The majority of commercial beekeepers who chauffeur their tiny workers from one state to another are hyper-vigilant about making sure the honeybees have food, water, and a temperature-controlled environment while they are on the trucks (as well as on the ground).

**

Before I began my enforced MS sojourn, I used to fly thousands of miles each and every year. Whether it was to Buenos Aires or Bologna, Katmandu or Crete, New Delhi or Dublin or Toronto or Tokyo, I loved visiting far-flung locales for both business and pleasure. Fortunately, I never had a single unsavory travel experience; my luggage was never lost, my flights were never cancelled, and I was never forced to white-knuckle my way through frightening high-altitude atmospheric turbulence. I had logged countless miles on the now-defunct Pan Am Airlines, and was always ready for a new travel adventure.

Today, when I spend close to 20 hours each day either sitting or lying in a recliner, I can't help but look back on those amazing long-ago trips with equal parts nostalgia and gratitude. MS definitely put a full-stop closure to my physically-active globe-trotting wanderlust ways.

Several years ago, Dr. James Levine, director of the Mayo Clinic at Arizona State University, decreed that *"Sitting is the new smoking,"* which naturally dismayed those of us with enforced stay-at-home lifestyles due to severe mobility challenges. Of course, his remarks were directed at the sedentary Americans who CHOOSE to sit for close to twelve hours each day, but for those of us who have no options whatsoever about our body's movement issues, it was yet another bit of unwelcome news…

***

As an antidote to all the migratory stressors, once the honeybees have finally completed their long-distance moving pollination services, as many as one third of commercial beekeepers bring their colonies to USDA Conservation Reserve Program (CRP) properties in the northern Great Plains. There are close to 30 million acres of available land that has plenty of forage, a minimum of pesticide exposure, and the welcomed and much-needed chance for the hard-working honeybees to rest and recover from their arduous travels.

While I was researching the long-distance itineraries of the countless female honeybees that pollinate America's crops, I couldn't help but acknowledge my schizophrenic reaction to their indentured mobility. On one hand, I worried about their forced-labor assignments, and the physical stressors that they endured while traveling. But the other part of me (the part that has a bad case of MS mandated cabin fever) envied the scenic upside they enjoyed as they repeatedly changed vistas and states and crops.

***

By the time I started writing this chapter, I had been receiving weekly BVT for three years. The honeybee stings still hurt, but I was more than willing to put up with the discomfort because I could honestly feel that my health was slowly—very slowly—improving. So, I was caught off guard one afternoon when a concerned and skeptical friend asked, *"But Marilyn, do you really think you're getting better?"*

I knew that the people in my life, particularly those who had read Pat Wagner's 1994 book *How Well Are You Willing To Bee?: A Beginner's "Auto" Fix It Guide*, were getting impatient over the fact that neither my mobility nor my independence had yet returned. The bee stings had ended Pat Wagner's days of being bedridden, and she regained the ability to live a "normal" life. But, unlike the Doubting Thomases in my life, I recognized that her astonishingly successful MS journey and mine had a number of major differences.

While (unlike me) Pat had been bedridden at one point, she began receiving BVT within a decade of her diagnosis, whereas mine didn't start until I'd had MS for 35 years. Plus, she was in her 30s when she began BVT, but my journey didn't start until I was 70 years old. And while she received 35 stings three times a week, Michael gave me 50 stings every seven days. Additionally, as we all know only too well, every case of MS is unique and different. So while the Stubborn Optimist in me *hoped* that I might one day be able to walk again, my more clear-headed goal was to simply stop the supposedly "inevitable" downward trajectory that was considered to be an unpleasant but irrefutable component of this dreadful disease.

My internal response to that friend's unexpected query was to make a mental list of the subtle (but positive) changes that I had noticed during the past 36 months. This is what I came up with:

VISUAL: This was perhaps the easiest category to measure because it was the most obvious. Without a doubt, since my bee stings had started, the appearance of my complexion, hair, and nails had all improved. As I mentioned earlier, I'd stopped losing hair, my fingernails no longer peeled or split, and many of my fine wrinkles seemed much less noticeable—to me as well as to others. On several occasions, my spirits have been lifted when people who haven't seen me for several years tell me that I look measurably healthier (i.e., better) than I used to.

For example, after one of my favorite couples had stopped by for a short Saturday afternoon visit, on their drive home, my girlfriend's husband commented to her (and this is a pretty unusual event coming from a guy) that he thought my hair had never looked so thick and shiny. Once she arrived home, she could hardly wait to call me and share that unexpected—if second-handed—honeybee-centric compliment.

Another undeniable benefit of the BVT sessions was that—ever since I'd lost the ability to walk—my ankles had turned into what was jokingly referred to as "cankles," which is officially described as "unusually thick or stout ankles." While there was minor physical discomfort connected to my swollen lower legs, I used to find it annoying that (from the knees down) I was a woman in her 40s who looked positively geriatric. Now, Michael gives me three stings around each ankle bone, and they look much less swollen and more defined…almost the way they used to before MS changed everything. Today, my ankles may not be exactly slender, but (hooray!) at least they no longer look like a medical textbook illustration of edema.

PHYSICAL: One of the most annoying "side effects" of having MS can be reoccurring (and particularly uncomfortable) UTI infections. In my case, for several decades, it seemed as if every four or five months I would be forced to take a course of antibiotics, which—knowing what they did to my biome in general—was something I truly dreaded. But ever since that very first bee sting, the unpleasant UTI issues have (miraculously) become a thing of the past. During the last three years (!), I've had neither a single antibiotic nor an annoying UTI infection.

Another welcome improvement has been the dramatic reduction in leg muscle cramps and spasms. It is annoying and painful to have a "Charley Horse," but be unable to stretch or "walk off" the discomfort. Where I once used to deal with these unwelcome visitors several times each day, they now rarely happen more than—at most—once a month.

Also, for decades, I had to use a straw any time I wanted to take a drink of water or coffee because (due to the tremor and slight weakness in my left hand) I was unable to safely lift a glass or a mug. As a result, my efforts to try and bring a beverage to my lips was often a messy challenge. But I was recently able to surprise my friends at a luncheon when I was—slowly but successfully—able to smoothly lift a coffee cup for a (very normal) sip. They were amazed that I didn't spill a single drop, and that I didn't have to rely on a straw. It's a small step, but it's the type of progress that a person coping with paralysis can't help but consider a major victory. There's no doubt in my mind that I have the honeybees (and their beneficial venom) to thank.

Additionally, I've received positive feedback from my talented physical therapists, who have commented that my limbs are far less stiff and rigid than they used to be. During my Monday morning appointments, I can now use the stationary NuStep bicycle far more energetically than I used to. As I mentioned earlier, when I first started my PT appointments, I could only complete five minutes at level one, but now I routinely finish over 20 minutes at level six. Again, even other professionals who have worked with MS patients are surprised to see these small, unconventional, but "inexplicable" signs of physical improvement.

EMOTIONAL: In her admirably honest best-selling book, *Mean Baby: A Memoir of Growing Up,* actress Selma Blair writes about her difficult struggles with MS. One of her poignant observations is that people who are coping with Multiple Sclerosis spend way too much time at home alone. I am aware of countless reasons for an MS patient's individual bouts of isolation—lack of access to caregivers, mobility challenges that range from stairs to curbs to "wheelchair hostile" destinations, issues regarding affordable transportation, the expense of being dependent on paid helpers, and the awkwardness of often being the only "disabled" person in the room.

I definitely experienced what Selma had observed during my first two decades with MS, but during the last three years I've noticed a dramatic uptick in my social life. It has gradually become easier to get dressed, less of a hassle to join others for lunch or a meeting, and—even in the midst of COVID-19—I now have the physical stamina to be "out and about" for far more hours in a day than I ever could before the honeybees became an essential and vital part of my life.

The emotional benefit of no longer feeling chronically isolated because of my wheelchair and MS has been positive on a variety of levels. For the first time in years, thanks to the BVT, I no longer feel cut off from the rest of the world simply because my body has been at war with a cruel and capricious autoimmune disease.

So, *"Yes, my friend, I am (slowly but surely) getting better…*

WHAT THE HONEYBEES TAUGHT ME

- The always-on-the-move traveling honeybees—who are forced to feed on a single food source for every crop they visit—would surely agree with British Romantic poet William Cowper (1730-1800), who believed that *"Variety is the spice of life."* After all, eating too much of only one thing (as in a mono diet) can be dangerous, dull, and unhealthy.

- It doesn't take long for the indentured traveling honeybees (and those who depend on their pollination services) to learn that all work and no play is ultimately dangerous, as well as expensive.

- Neither people nor *Apis mellifera* have the ability to always choose precisely where, when, for whom (or why) they work.

- Depending on your perspective, sometimes tiny baby steps can actually feel like triumphant strides made in Seven-League Boots.

- Anthony Bourdain (1956-2018) must have had the indentured honeybees in mind when he wrote, *"Travel isn't always pretty. It isn't always comfortable. Sometimes it hurts, it even breaks your heart. But that's okay. The journey changes you; it should change you.... You take something with you. Hopefully, you leave something good behind."*

Chapter 12
Apitherapy

The first wealth is health.
Ralph Waldo Emerson (1803-1882)

Christopher Reeve, the much-admired star of *Superman,* was a hero to millions of people for a variety of worthwhile reasons. Back in 2004, only a few months before he died, I was lucky enough to meet and interview him. Seated side-by-side and motionless in our black vinyl wheelchairs, we made a strange-looking couple.

His riding accident had left him a quadriplegic, and his gigantic, motorized wheelchair—ideal for his six-foot-four frame—towered over my smaller and petite vinyl one. We could not have been more different physically (I am five foot six, and can still use my left arm, while he was totally paralyzed and dependent on a rotating staff of caregivers, as well as the occasional use of a ventilator.) Plus, he was an award-winning, genuinely handsome, world-famous movie star, with incredibly intense blue eyes, and I was, well, me.

Despite our physical and professional differences, we did have our respective and unique disabilities in common, Superman and I quickly bonded over our shared paralysis-enforced challenges. Like me, he was struggling to escape an enforced new reality that had changed every single aspect of his life. When it was finally time for me to leave, he turned his brilliant blue eyes my way, and practically commanded me to remember: *"Marilyn, keep searching for your cure. Once you have decided to choose hope, anything is possible."*

There is no doubt in my mind that those four letters—h.o.p.e.—are the reason that I became a Bee Geek back in 2019. Up until that point, I was living in a world of unrequited Stubborn Optimism in which every authorized medical voice I heard insisted that those of us with MS could only expect to get more (and more) ill. The memory of annoyed and irritated neurologists (with the exception of Dr. David Perlmutter) who shook their heads at my quest for something—anything—that might improve my situation is forever seared in my battered memory bank.

When I initially learned that the ancient Egyptians and Chinese effectively used apitherapy (defined as *The medicinal use of products that are being made and produced by honeybees*), I began to research *Apis mellifera* health-enhancing treatments in earnest. I learned that Hippocrates, who has long been considered the Father of Medicine, used "bee products" to treat both arthritis and joint pain. And by the 1800s, European doctors were conducting clinical studies to validate bee venom's positive effect on rheumatism.

***

It's important to remember that apitherapy is a broad term that includes a variety of different beneficial modalities. Essentially, many different honeybee products, including bee air, beeswax, honeycomb, pollen, propolis, raw honey and royal jelly, can play a subtle but significant role in improving health and wellbeing.

As I've mentioned before, the beekeepers I've come to know and respect all have one trait in common: They rarely agree with each other about anything regarding *Apis mellifera*. One beekeeper will swear that sugar water increases his hives' honey output, while another will say that sugar water is a deceitful way of tricking bees into working even harder than they already do, and a third will say that human dietary "assistance" interferes with the ancient and natural order of beekeeping. Because I am genetically conflict-adverse, and more of a suburban-honeybee observer than a caregiver, I'm happy to listen to their opinions, but I rarely express one of my own.

And while their positions regarding the care and feeding and supervision of their hives may differ, when it comes to the topic of apitherapy every beekeeper has plenty to say, most of which disagrees with their colleagues' opinions. A South Florida female beekeeper who is also an apitherapist, recently shared photos of a breast cancer survivor whose "lump" disappeared after receiving hundreds of localized stings. A fellow apitherapist, however, disagreed and argued that he didn't believe it was possible to remove a tumor with bee venom. He did, however, insist that very few beekeepers die of cancer because the bee stings are so beneficial to the immune system. And almost every beekeeper and apitherapist I've ever met (or read about) will happily share stories about people they've treated who have recovered from Lyme disease, eliminated arthritis, improved Type 2 diabetes, and managed a host of other unwelcomed conditions after using bees to boost their overall well being.

In today's world, people appear to be slightly more open to alternative medicine than they used to be, but there's nothing "new and improved" about using bee products for medicinal purposes. In fact, thousands of years ago various far-flung cultures (such as the Chinese, Egyptian, Greek, and Russian) used bee products for their healing qualities. Practically everything associated with honeybees—from beehive air to bee venom to beeswax to pollen, propolis, raw honey and royal jelly—eventually became part of healers' arsenal to improve health and fight diseases.

In twelfth-century Syria, *The Book of Medicines*, included over 1,000 prescriptions, and over 350 of them required the use of bee products for their healing properties. And going back even farther, to third-century B.C. China, the Hunan Province's book of 52 medicinal prescriptions included several that relied on bee products. The Ancient Egyptians routinely used apitherapy products to combat arthritis, digestive ailments, rheumatism, and a variety of other health issues.

Currently, where double-blind medical studies (a type of clinical trial in which neither the participants nor the researchers know which treatment or intervention is being used until the clinical trial is over.) are the norm, apitherapy is considered by many to be an under-documented branch of alternative medicine. An entire book could be written about any of the following bee products, but I've chosen instead to give you a brief introduction to these alternative healing options.

BEEHIVE AIR:

In Central European countries (Austria, Germany, Hungary, Lithuania, Slovenia, and Ukraine), beehive air therapy is used for anti-aging, beauty, pulmonary conditions, and other medicinal purposes. The idea is for humans to breathe the same air that the bees do in order to boost immunity and initiate feelings of general well-being.

Until I'd received more than a year's worth of stings, I'd never heard of beehive air as a complementary component of apitherapy. But Professor Stashenko invited me to experience his customized backyard beehive air sanctuary. My favorite Ukrainian beekeeper had placed a 20-foot-travel trailer on top of 17 active screened-off beehives. Each white wooden box contained about 60,000 bees, so while sitting inside the trailer I was essentially sharing the same atmosphere as over one million hard-working honeybees. The impact of a one-hour session (essentially, a short time-out nap) was gentle and soothing; by my third session, I noticed that while I'd arrived feeling frazzled and slightly grumpy, I left the trailer with a pronounced sense of calm. I felt clear, focused, refreshed, and in a measurably-improved mood.

A 2018 Bee Research Department Study by the Egyptian Agricultural Research Centre studied the antibacterial, anti-inflammatory, and antiviral properties in connection with the chemical composition of beehive air. Fifty-six different volatiles were identified, which helps explain why people feel that their overall well-being is enhanced when they breathe beehive air.

This alternative modality has been frequently used to treat respiration tract disorders (asthma, bronchitis, lung fibrosis, etc.) as well as a way to alleviate depression. An apitherapist in Spain recently posted online that his beehive air was responsible for a positive effect on a patient suffering from Parkinson's.

Those mysterious honeybee pheromones—in addition to the subtle vibrations form the hive—are considered to be beneficial to human health in general, but apitherapists are still researching these topics.

BEESWAX:

While beeswax has traditionally been thought to remedy a variety of dermatological issues (as we discussed in Chapter 5), it is not just a building component for honey and larvae storage. Humans have relied on beeswax for centuries, and its popularity shows no signs of slowing down. In his book *How to Use Beeswax and Honey to Cure Skin Problems*, Gene Ashburner argued that because of its emollient and vitamin A content, beeswax can also assist with cellular reconstruction while it simultaneously locks in moisture and softens dry skin without clogging pores.

A 2013 study in the *Korean Journal of Internal Medicine* found that various antioxidant alcohols found in honeycomb were also beneficial to liver function. The components of beeswax appear to also lower the bloodstream's "bad" (LDL) cholesterol while raising "good" HDL cholesterol levels. Since beeswax is antibacterial and anti-inflammatory, it can actually benefit a variety of dermatological issues ranging from acne to arthritis swelling to "jock itch".

As we discussed in Chapter 5, beeswax is created by very young bees who secrete small slivers of wax from special glands in their abdomen. The young worker bees combine nectar and honey into a compound that includes carbon, hydrogen, and oxygen; this is what's used to construct the honeycomb structure that houses larva and honey within the hive. It takes six pounds of honey for the worker bees to create only one pound of beeswax.

The accumulation of beeswax is a laborious process that involves the bee using her legs to move the small deposit of wax to her mouth, where she uses her tongue to turn it into a string or ribbon of wax that's combined with a liquid to give the substance a sticky nature. With the help of other bees, a block of wax is created that will very quickly be turned into honeycomb; in the course of a full year a strong hive can create as much as 15 pounds of beeswax, which can be used cosmetically or medicinally.

As of this writing, there is no scientific way to replicate beeswax. It is composed of close to 300 different trace quantities of compounds, including esters, free fatty acids, minerals, acids, and alcohols. Today, beeswax is an essential component of a wide variety of modern creams, masks, ointments, patches, and suppositories. As long ago as 400 B.C, Hippocrates recommended applying beeswax on the neck to treat throat pain and tonsillitis. During that same era, a mixture of beeswax and olive oil was the standard topical treatment for bone fractures.

Beeswax is considered useful for all skin conditions including burns, frostbite, ulcers and wounds because it simultaneously protects skin and stimulates tissue growth. One of my local bee experts insists that chewing honeycomb (i.e., beeswax) is a great way to protect tooth enamel, strengthen gums, as well as treat hay fever. And when applied topically, beeswax can accelerate the normal healing time of bruises and burns.

Beeswax is an essential ingredient in "moist exposed burn ointment" (MEBO), which has been used in China on over half a million patients to reduce burn victims' healing time and length of hospitalization. This is an important advancement because 70% of all burn victims who die in the US do so because of infections, and bee products are unsurpassed when it comes to its ability to fight bacteria.

In addition to its role in dentistry and orthodontic procedures, liquified beeswax has also been used to reduce pain in afflicted arthritic joints.

BEE VENOM:

The Chinese have used honeybees to sting people on acupuncture points for over 3,000 years, but it wasn't until the 1800s that the use of bee venom was introduced to modern European cultures. Back in 1888, Austrian physician Philip Terc (1844-1917) wrote about his success treating rheumatism patients with bee venom. BVT (bee venom therapy) is the use of live bee stings to treat a variety of challenging physical problems that include arthritis, carpal tunnel syndrome, low back pain, lupus, MS, shingles, tennis elbow, and varicose veins. For an amazing look at what happens if you get stung by a honeybee, make sure to log onto this astonishing YouTube video: https://www.youtube.com/watch?v=IzVe3lyf4Fg.

The reason bee venom is so effective for such a wide variety of physical issues is that it produces an immediate anti-inflammatory response without negatively affecting the body's immune system. Some people refer to this as "Bee-acupuncture" or "acupuncture on steroids" because the stings are applied on specific meridians.

In the 1920s, Dr. Bodog Beck's book *Bee Venom Therapy* inspired several American doctors (primarily in Hollywood, Connecticut, and Vermont) to continue his work. His remarkable success with arthritis patients had earned him the nickname of "King of BVT."

For people like me (who live with a variety of chronic MS symptoms), the primary beneficial ingredient in bee venom is Apamin, which affects the electrical signals that have been blocked by nerve sheath degeneration. Many people in the health field believe that all illness stems from toxic levels of inflammation, and bee venom—in addition to being anti-bacterial and anti-viral—has strong anti-inflammatory properties as well.

It's important to remember that bee venom doesn't really "cure" anything; instead, it triggers the body's immune system into action to heal itself. Some people feel this is because BVT stimulates the adrenal glands to produce more Cortisol, which is our body's natural non-toxic form of Cortisone. A bee sting will cause a small area to turn red and swell, which brings fluid to the area that washes away toxins; the new blood that arrives stimulates an itching sensation. That unpleasant heat, the swelling, and itchy feelings are signals to us that the bee venom is doing its job.

Thousands of people on a health quest put up with the discomfort of bee stings because they feel it helps their specific physical problem, and—as a bonus—it also serves as an effective immune system booster. Full disclosure: For a few minutes, the stings can really hurt. And, depending upon how many stings you receive, the aftereffect can feel like a mild case of the flu.

Currently, about 5% of the American population is actively allergic to bee venom, which means they will go into anaphylactic shock if stung. For the rest of us, it takes about ten stings per pound of body weight to be deadly. I weigh 125 pounds, and receive about 50 stings each week, I'm not afraid of the stings; instead, I concentrate on simply improving my health profile, even if the process is slower than I would like.

POLLEN:

The foraging bees that gather nectar (the raw component destined to become honey) return to the hive with pollen that is in their leg pouches (the corbiculae), and has stuck to their bodies. The various pollens that they bring back contain a variety of essential amino acids, which are molecules that combine to form proteins. Essentially, amino acids and proteins are the tiny—but essential—building blocks of life, and the pollen that honeybees bring back to the hive actually contain more of these essential amino acids than milk (Got Pollen?).

According to French Honorary Sorbonne Professor Emeritus Remy Chauvin (1913-2009), pollen also contains important fatty acids that help reduce cholesterol levels and contribute to cell regeneration. Additionally, pollen serves as an effective detoxifier because of its antibacterial, antioxidant, antiviral effect. My local beekeepers may disagree about many aspects of the honeybee world, but they all insist that taking pollen on a regular basis should be considered an essential part of conscientious self-care.

PROPOLIS:

Often referred to as "bee glue," propolis is a plant-derived natural substance that the honeybees collect from trees and plants. Because it contains a variety of valuable polyphenols, propolis is frequently used as a construction component inside beehive or nests.

When it comes to human consumption, however, propolis is a highly effective antioxidant and free radical scavenger. Many beekeepers believe that propolis protects against cardiovascular disease and increases longevity; its positive effect on brain tissue has made it of particular interest to researchers working on Alzheimer's, MS, and Parkinson's. Because of its powerful role in vasodilation, there have also been suggestions that propolis can be useful as a preventative treatment for both myopia and macular degeneration.

RAW HONEY:

Do you remember "Gus Portokalos," the father in the 2002 hit movie *My Big Fat Greek Wedding*? His firm belief that Windex was able to solve or fix every household problem always made the audience laugh. Well, ever since I've been a resident in the honeybee universe, I've met a variety of beekeepers who feel exactly the same way about the miraculous qualities of raw honey.

From boosting energy, to eliminating acne, fighting allergies, treating gingivitis, improving the digestive tract, eliminating skin infections, healing wounds (without creating a scar), lowering Type 2 Diabetics' plasma glucose levels, preventing bladder infections, and soothing sore throats, chances are your local beekeeper will automatically recommend using raw honey rather than relying on a commercial pharmaceutical product.

Its important to understand that buying a container of honey from a big box or a local grocery store is not your best option, Why? Because that level of "pure" or "organic" honey has probably been either adulterated with chemical additives or (even more likely) has been "over processed."

Instead, buying honey from a local beekeeper will ensure that it is raw (i.e. unheated) and full of beneficial locally-derived nectar and pollen. For the last four years, I've purchased countless half-gallon jugs of the Professor's home-harvested honey, and I wouldn't consider using anything else for either edible or topical apitherapy purposes. I've also discovered that this sort of local pure raw honey makes a much-appreciated gift for family and friends.

ROYAL JELLY:

In Hollywood, during the 1950s, Royal Jelly was considered to be the most-effective highest-quality skin care ingredient available. Back then at least, half a dozen different American cosmetics companies sold face creams that contained Royal Jelly, which had been added to their other ingredients.

At the beginning of the last century, French doctor Leonard Bordas (1880-1962) began analyzing what made Royal Jelly so potent. Why do the drones and worker bees (who only receive Royal Jelly for the first three days of their lives) live for only six short weeks, but the Queens (who never eat anything other than Royal Jelly) live for six whole years?

The mysterious thick yellowish cream-like substance is only produced by the youngest worker bees, and it—inexplicably—actually has an amino acid component that is similar (but also superior) to the protein found in eggs, meat, and milk.

Unfortunately, Royal Jelly oxidizes quickly, so it has a minimal shelf life unless it undergoes a process known as **Lyophilization**. This is similar (but superior) to what most of us know as freeze drying. This link (CN102670730B - Process for producing royal jelly extract lyophilized powder - Google Patents) will explain why this process maintains the viability of Royal Jelly, which would otherwise have a very short shelf life.

The combination of enzymes, hormones, and vitamins makes it a nutrient powerhouse for bees, and a useful ingredient for cosmetics. When it comes to medicinal purposes, proponents will argue that it does everything from burn adipose tissue to improve immunity to stimulate appetite, and increase muscle strength.

WHAT THE HONEYBEES TAUGHT ME

- All bee-related activities were considered so therapeutic for returning WWI soldiers that (in 1919) the Federal Board for Vocational Education sponsored "Uncle Sam Foots the Bill." It was a subsidized beekeeping program designed to help counteract the brutal effects of war. Essentially, honeybee hives were the first iteration of PTSD therapy.

- Sara George wrote a wonderful novel (*The Beekeeper's Pupil*) in 2002 about Francois Huber (1750-1831), the blind French naturalist who made the study of bees his life's work. As if speaking on behalf of the wise and health-giving honeybees, Huber's assistant soon discovers that "Every sting makes us stronger."

- While talking with beekeepers who were more than happy to share their first-hand healing stories, I attained a higher degree of medical open-mindedness. Thanks to the honeybees, I learned to cautiously embrace **heterodoxy** (i.e., not conforming with accepted or orthodox standards or beliefs.) when it comes to physical health.

- Frequently, there is a huge chasm between things that might be considered superficial (i.e., how we look) from those that are essential (i.e., how healthy we are). But in the honeybee world, it's all considered to be one and the same thanks to their ability to make everything—from the superficial to the essential— better.

- During my almost four-decade struggle with MS, I've tried to remember the words of Hippocrates (375 B.C. -460 B.C.) who believed that *Healing is a matter of time, but it is sometimes a matter of opportunity.* It took me a long time—and many false starts—before the honeybees and I were able to work together. That prolonged search taught me to embrace a new form of patience, and has made a tremendous difference in both my mental and physical well-being.

Chapter 13
Honeybee Dangers

To be the equal of reality you must learn how to
ignore it without danger.
Lawrence Durrell (1912-1990)

COVID-19, food shortages, global warming, political instability, terrorism, the war in Ukraine, and countless other negative contemporary factors are issues that currently—and continually—threaten our *homo sapien* increasingly fragile peace of mind.

During my years of honeybee immersion, I learned that *Apis mellifera* has also faced equally daunting additional challenges. For millennia, honeybees have managed to survive a wide variety of potential dangers from aggressive animals (think bears and skunks), chemicals, Colony Collapse Disorder (CCD), humans, other hostile insects, poor nutrition, and even Mother Nature herself.

***

As a child, my anxieties were focused on youthful worries and simple concerns that included: homework assignments, music lessons and performances, the perpetual "relocations" our little family endured, and the fear that accompanied my never-ending "new girl" status at school. In retrospect, those seem like genuinely juvenile "problems" because even though they felt ominous and painful at the time, the truth is that—as a youngster—I really didn't have any truly serious worries.

Fortunately, my parents saw to it that all my physical and educational needs were met, so I was able to fall asleep each night secure in the knowledge that I was loved—even if I didn't have a clue about (or the ability to control) what life might be like in the next town or at the next school.

When I became a parent, however, it felt as if the number of life's "scary situations" grew exponentially. I worried about my little boys' health and wellbeing, my perpetually inadequate bank balance, the continual challenges of household expenses and maintenance (i.e., the moist basement, the leaky roof, the aging fireplace, the never-ending tax bills (state, federal, property, etc.), as well as the challenges of meeting my editors' and publishers' expectations.

After MS arrived, I was given an unwanted front-row seat that (unfortunately) helped put my earlier school girl fears in perspective. With the benefit of a hard-won hindsight, I was finally able to see how truly inconsequential those other long-ago imagined and youthful so-called dangers had been.

During the decades of my young adulthood, when I felt that each day brought new things to worry about, I longed to be like my two favorite female TV characters. With every fiber of my high-strung tightly-wound self, I wanted to exude the calm, elegant, graceful yet strong mindset of Lady Marjorie from the BBC's classic five-season drama *Upstairs,*

Downstairs. And during the roller-coaster years when my young sons and I would watch *Little House on the Prairie* together, I really (*really*) wanted to be as kind and gentle and sweet as Caroline Ingalls; as you can imagine, neither of those role-model wishes were ever fulfilled.

So, the only solution for a frazzled single mom in the late 1970's was to "*Do whatever it takes*," and meet each challenge that surfaced to the best of my stumbling non-thespian ability. Desperate times, of course, all-too-often call for desperate measures, and when they have been overpowered by fear, actress-inspired coping mechanisms are often inadequate. That is when grace and elegance are forced to assume other–far more practical—forms of expression.

***

When I remembered all the outside forces that had impacted my hyper-stressful earlier life, it ignited my curiosity to look more closely at the honeybee population. I wanted to closely examine the various negative factors that threaten its well-being. Below is a short list of what I learned about *Apis mellifera* dangers:

Colony Collapse Disorder (CCD): This beekeeping problem is a mystery that has spawned as many different theories as the 1963 assassination of JFK. In human terms, CCD would essentially be like a huge condominium complex in which—literally overnight—all the adults inexplicably disappeared, but the infants and children were left behind, abandoned, and unattended. I've been told that opening a hive that has suffered CCD can be spooky because the only adult bee that remains with the abandoned beeswax, brood, and honey is the lifeless body of the heartbroken dead Queen.

Many unproven theories have tried to explain why thousands of honeybees seem to simply "evaporate," including everything from disorienting cellphone vibrations to toxic airplane emissions to societal events, to inexplicable intergalactic signals.

The bad news is that thousands of hives have been affected. The good news, however, is that because of CCD's mysterious status millions of people around the globe have finally how finally begun to recognize just how essential and fragile honeybees are.

During the last 30 years, global awareness of how vitally important bees are to human life, how psychologically delicate these little insects are, and how challenging it is to counteract the myriad dangers that the honeybees face each day on every single continent, has skyrocketed.

Chemicals: Common pesticides (like mosquito sprays) present a particular challenge because foraging honeybees can accidentally bring topical poisons back to the hives. When aerial spraying is scheduled (as it was during the Zika outbreak) some beekeepers have a warning system that alerts them so they can cover their hives with old parachute fabric to prevent the poisonous mist from killing their honeybees. Even the use of residential pesticides by gardeners and landscapers can present a serious threat; one local suburban beekeeper (who is a good friend) lost six entire hives overnight because a neighbor's yard was accidentally "over sprayed."

Among the biggest chemical threats to honeybees is the use of neonicotinoids, which is a group of insecticides used widely on farms and in urban landscapes. When sprayed, they are absorbed by plants, and can be present in flowers, nectar, and well as pollen.

As of 2013, neonicotinoids were used on about 95% of corn and canola crops, on most cotton, sorghum, and sugar beet fields, on about half of all domestic soybean crops, as well as on many fruit, vegetable, and grain harvests. These powerful insecticides have shown increased mortality rates in honeybees, as well as serious sublethal effects. They can damage delicate wing tissue, as well as the bees' ability to effectively fly, forage, and navigate.

A 2017 international survey discovered evidence of neonicotinoids in over 70% of honey samples, which illustrates just how pervasive and difficult to control these insecticides have become. As a result, the Environmental Protection Agency has established three separate "categories" for pesticides. Those that are harmful to bees are listed as Category 1, and they are required to have a warning label. Those products are ones that can potentially harm aquatic life, bees, birds, and a variety of mammals.

Deformed Wing Virus: This cruel illness destroys the honeybee's ability to fly. It prevents an infected larvae from developing normal wings; as a result, the newborn honeybee emerges with wings that appear either melted or shriveled in size. Since those birth-defect bees cannot contribute to the hive's well-being, death is inevitable. Mites also spread Acute Bee Paralysis, which is another deadly infection that can threaten the hive.

Meteorological Instability: Climate change is another "natural" threat to *Apis mellifera*. According to the Honeybee Research and Extension Laboratory at the University of Florida, weather is among the top five killers of honeybees in America. Frigidity in the North, drought in the West, extreme heat and flooding in the South and South East—not to mention the hurricanes we experience here in Florida—all present a serious danger to honeybees.

In September of 2022, Florida beekeepers learned first-hand just how cruel Mother Nature can be when Hurricane Ian battered the state. Florida's normal beehive population hovers around 800,000; 60% of which are professional pollinators. Ian was a Category 4 Storm that had sustained winds of over 150 miles per hour. As a result it will take years to rebuild Florida's beekeeping industry. The impact will be felt by almond growers in California, in apple and pear orchards in the Pacific Northwest, and even among blueberry and cranberry growers in New England.

Tracheal Mite: This miniscule pest is about the size of a dust speck, and it invades and infects the honeybees' airways. Sadly, of course, the list of "natural" predators goes on and on and on.

Varroa mites: Ever since 2007, the Bee Informed Partnership has conducted an annual

National Colony Loss and Management Survey to measure bee-related risk factors and protective approaches connected to beekeeping. According to the study, from April 2020 to April 2021 beekeepers lost over 45% of their managed honeybee colonies. This is, of course, an alarming threat to bees (as well as to all of humanity). This miniscule extremely dangerous insect literally feeds on *Apis mellifera*, and also transmits deadly viruses to bees.

From 1980 until the late 90s, those tiny Varroa (or vampire) mites seriously damaged the international beekeeping industry. The female mites lay their eggs inside the hives' brood cells; they also cling to the adult honeybees, and then (literally) suck out the bees' blood, which is their preferred source of nutrients.

Remember how I mentioned earlier that beekeepers rarely agree on anything regarding their hives? The topic of fighting mites is a perfect example of differing opinions; many beekeepers try to eliminate the Varroa threat by regularly using pesticides, while others argue that mite-killing chemicals can also damage or kill honeybees. This "hands-off" approach, however, carries its own dangers because those murderous little parasites can quickly overtake and destroy countless hives.

Part of what makes Varroa so dangerous is the hyper-invasive way it multiplies once it's inside the hive. After a mite climbs into the hexagonal brood chamber, it hides until the honeycomb is "capped," with a nutrient-rich toping. Instead of only attacking adult honeybees, Varroa actually prefer to stealthily enter the cell, and then hide underneath the five-day old larvae that are 24 hours away from being capped. Three days later, the adult female mite will lay her first egg, which will be male. After that, she will then lay a female egg every 30 hours. It only takes six days for all of those newborn mites to reach sexual maturity and (yikes!) begin the reproductive process all over again. This results in catastrophic damage to any emerging honeybees. The mites are also dangerous because they can transmit other deadly diseases as well.

Vespa Hornets: These insects pose one of the major threats to hives because they are both large (about the size of a matchbox) and bloodthirsty (they enter a hive, decapitate the bees, and then take the headless bodies back to serve as a meal for their offspring).

As we know, honeybees are so obsessive about cleanliness that they always "wait" or leave the safety of their hive or nest rather than "relieve themselves" inside. But Heather Mattila (of Wellesley College) discovered that bees in Vietnam incorporated using other animals' feces at the entrance of their hives. As I mentioned earlier, the bees would gather small bits of odiferous excrement from various farm animals (think chickens, cows, goats, and pigs) and then place the tiny clumps around the entrance to their nest. As a result (because of the noxious smell), the hostile hornets spend less time trying to enter the hives.

Wax Moth: This is another insect that has a unique battle plan that can seriously harm a hive. They commandeer the honeycomb environment to serve as a stolen nursery for their own offspring. The cream-colored larvae of this insect then create twisted tunnels in the beeswax, which destroys the standard hexagonal cells that are essential to a healthy honeybee community. After the wax moths emerge as a living pale enemy, they essentially have the ability to turn honeycomb into worthless brown crumbles. Another unwelcome insect is the **Small Hive Beetle**, which is only one-third the size of a worker bee, and has a dark and hard protective covering that the honey bees' stingers cannot penetrate.

The good news is that a biotech company (Dalan Animal Health) in Athens, Georgia, has received conditional approval from the US Department of Agriculture for a potential honeybee vaccine. The vaccine, which contains dead versions of the *Paenibacillus larvae* bacterium, will be incorporated into Royal Jelly, and then fed to their Queen Bee. Once the vaccine exists inside her ovaries, all her offspring will enjoy immunity from a variety of diseases.

During my research, I discovered a honeybee threat that actually had links to the insanity of Adolf Hitler's Nazi Germany. In 2018, in the Austrian state of Carinthia, a successful beekeeper was penalized because his docile but hard-working bees were considered "too dark." He was ordered by officials to replace his Queens (who were judged to be "leather brown-orange") with ones that were "light gray." The beekeeper refused the order, and labelled it "racial fanaticism."

The dispute is over whether or not the strain of "true Carniolan" bees was being diluted by honeybees from non-Austrian *Apis mellifera*. Fines for keepers with "mixed" hives can run as high as $6,000, and some hardliners have tried to push for uncooperative beekeepers to be given prison sentences. It's sad to think that with all of the other dangers that honeybees face, there version of skin color has become an issue!

***

Just when I began to get deeply ensconced regarding all the various problems that *Apis mellifera* faced, I learned about yet another amazing contribution that these remarkable insects make to improve the human experience. You may remember the Nicholas Sparks' 1995 bestselling book *The Horse Whisperer,* which was made into a hit 1998 movie that starred Robert Redford. But you probably didn't know (I certainly didn't) that there is a gifted scientist with a PhD in Entomology (he minored in Biochemistry and Philosophy) who has essentially been a "bee whisperer" for the past four decades.

He actually began his honeybee journey in a rather convoluted way. He wrote his PhD thesis on, the different noises that the Big-Headed Grasshopper makes, which eventually turned into an analysis of their "vocabulary" of sounds. Back in the 1970s, Bromenshenk worked with a team that had been assigned to measure the effect of coal-fired power plants on local insects in Montana, North Dakota and Wyoming. Over 5,000 bee colonies were monitored as part of his research project for the Environmental Protection Agency.

Dr. Jerry Bromenshenk is now retired from the University of Montana, but at one point he monitored millions of active honeybees for the EPD, and paid particular attention to every aspect of their behavior. Instead of working as a regular professor, which would have involved hours and hours of classroom responsibility, Dr. Bromenshenk became a grant-sponsored Research Professor. This allowed him to concentrate on environmental insect monitoring. Along with five other epidemiologist experts, he founded Bee Alert Technology, Inc., a company whose specialty is measuring the impact of toxic threats to *Apis mellifera*, as well as the environment.

He loved working with honeybees because (for his specialized scientific research purposes) they seemed like convenient "flying dust mops" whose tiny body hairs effortlessly picked up miniscule levels of airborne toxins. He was soon recruited to work at different government sites—from Puget Sound to variety of Department of Defense and US Army locations. Dr. Bromenshenk soon noticed that the sounds honeybees made changed whenever they were exposed to toxic chemicals—like the ones specifically found in plastic landmines.

While working with honeybees, he noticed that they were quickly able to identify and learn about their environment, even if it was on unstable and moving pontoon boats that were used as a base from which the bees could detect chemical explosives. In 2003, he and four other University of Montana faculty members created Bee Alert Technology, and in 2012 they introduced a hand-held device that was a first attempt to efficiently record and analyze *Apis mellifera* sounds.

By 2017, both Android and Apple began to offer smart phones with processors that could turn a job that use to take minutes into a seconds-only task, and as a result the Bee Health Guru app was born. This allows beekeepers anywhere in the world to track bee behavior and sounds. If you would like to learn more about this technology visit www.BeekeepingTodayPodcast.com

Currently, Dr. Bromenshenk and his team maintain around 50 honeybee colonies, and his Online Master Beekeeping Course is internationally available in over a dozen countries. Thanks to Dr. Bromenshenk and his bees, fields of dangerous landmines are safely being cleared, and hidden stores of toxic chemicals are being discovered and unearthed. Additionally, our understanding of bee behavior—as well as their various forms of auditory communication—are being identified, better understood, and shared with honeybee lovers everywhere.

***

I'm pretty sure that it would be very difficult for anyone to sit in a doctor's office and receive the devastating diagnosis of a "Chronic, incurable, progressive, neurological disease," and not be frightened. It's not easy to cope with all the conflicting and confusing emotions that arise when your own body—in the form of an autoimmune disease—begins to attack itself. In many ways, it feels like an incredibly cruel, dangerous, unwanted, and very hostile twist of fate.

When I first dealt with the harsh realities of living with MS, my fears were based on the unimaginable possibilities of never being able to dance, ride horses, or even walk again. At the time, I had no way of knowing that the realities of living in a wheelchair for decades would carry other challenges that would be far more potent and toxic than mere immobility.

In my case, I found it far easier to cope with uncooperative muscles than with the overwhelming and unrelenting presence of multi-faceted frustration "episodes" fueled by a body that refuses to obey the simplest of requests. Countless times, when I could no longer grip, hold, or successfully reach for something I needed or wanted to touch, the frightening reality of my profound dependency shattered both my heart and my fragile self-esteem.

I am not ashamed to admit that I am far more frightened of the **consequences** of being paralyzed than of the actual paralysis itself. I do an excellent job of masquerading my inner version of Edvard Munch's (1863-1944) *The Scream,* but the truth is that my meltdowns and tears are always way too close to the surface. I rarely—if ever—have the luxury of being able to (completely) emotionally "exhale."

Medical experts warn that those of us with MS face an extensive laundry list of potentially serious and unpleasant possibilities that can seem overwhelming. The "predicted" inescapable physical dangers can include the harmful consequences of getting overheated, the complications that accompany numbness and loss of feeling, scary infections, the restriction of normal vision or voice, as well as a lengthy list of nightmarish unsavory digestive issues. Sadly, the list goes on and on and on.

In all the thousands of pages I've read regarding MS—from individuals who've lived with it as well as those who treat it—there is rarely a whisper about the emotional side effects that surface countless times every single day. Mentally, the consequences of having MS can be brutal and, frankly, dangerous. I have lived with those hurtful feelings, and their lingering consequences for decades. Fortunately, those negative emotions come and go, and thanks to my Stubborn Optimism I have never totally lost hope or abandoned my belief in a natural-based treatment or (please, God) a cure.

Forty months after I first began to get my weekly bee stings, I sat in my recliner one night and watched my right big toe twitch uncontrollably for a full five minutes. It had been several decades since any part of that foot had been able to move on its own. I was, of course, surprised, encouraged, and overcome with joy at the mere possibility that (ahem) I had just witnessed a completely unexpected "Something Wonderful" episode. Small moments like that one, allow me to deal with the Matterhorn-sized accumulation of my daily MS battles with a slow-growing sense of confidence.

Danger has many definitions, and whether you are a honeybee or a woman who has been in a wheelchair for over three decades, emotional and intellectual coping skills are essential. It's a challenge that I work on every single day, and I truly believe that the vulnerable *Apis mellifera* is as determined and hopeful and persistent as I am…

WHAT THE HONEYBEES TAUGHT ME

- Female worker bees have a short (45 day) lifespan and face a wide variety of dangers without ever appearing frightened. Their unflinching focus on productivity rather than paranoia reminded me of media legend David Sarnoff's (1921-2017) advice, *"We cannot banish dangers, but we can banish fears. We must not demean life by standing in awe of death."*

- Just when I thought (about four years into my honeybee love affair) that I knew almost everything there was to know about *Apis mellifera*, I discovered that a remarkable researcher in Montana had made a discovery that even my over-active imagination could have never fathomed. Bottom line: No matter how much you think you know about honeybees, they will always surprise you. And they will do it in the most remarkable way…

- Learning that a dust speck-sized predator could wipe out an entire honeybee colony taught me that sometimes, (i.e., especially when we least expect it) what looks like a tiny issue can—if not adequately addressed—turn into a huge problem.

- Throughout the ages, honeybees have managed to survive every imaginable type of hostile environment, but the chemical assaults they have faced during the last century are the most dangerous threat they've ever encountered.

- In spite of the hostile and atmospheric perils they face, the bees continue to follow their inner programing as they wait for chemists and scientists to quit assaulting their environment. It's almost as if they agree with or understand the words of Max Planck (1858-1947), who was frustrated because the elderly change-resistant "experts" often ignored what was obvious, but too new to be accepted. He went on to win the 1918 Nobel prize in theoretical physics, and stated that *"Science progresses funeral by funeral."*

- I loved learning that *Apis mellifera* will never be fully domesticated, but they can (by using propolis or their stingers) manage to still effectively defend themselves. They have helped humans for thousands of years, but they will never stop demanding that we fully acknowledge how important it is to respect their autonomy.

Chapter 14
Apis mellifera's Famous Friends

There are certain pursuits which, if not wholly poetic and true, do at least suggest a nobler and finer relation to nature than we know. The keeping of bees, for instance.
Henry David Thoreau (1817-1862)

Until I became fascinated by all things honeybee, I had no idea that there were so many celebrities who share my newfound obsession. Just as I had learned while I researched household-name individuals with MS, it soon began to feel as if small-scale beekeeping has become an unexpected shared experience among many (past and present) A-listers.

During my years of interviewing and profiling celebrities for different newspaper and magazine articles, I'd had a front-row seat that helped me observe different popular and well-publicized trends. For example, in the 1980s, it felt as if every third actor or actress in Hollywood had begun chanting "*Nam myoho renge kyo*" on a regular basis. And, of course, we all remember the A-lister's devotion to gluten-free food and juice-fast regimens. Then, after COVID-19 struck, everyone from Hugh Jackman to Jimmy Fallon was proudly baking their own sourdough French bread. But the more I researched, the more I realized that—through the ages—keeping beehives had also become a far more mindful soothing and health-promoting activity than those other passing fads.

Due to my long-list of physical challenges, it never occurred to me to even consider having beehives of my own. After all, I need tons of help from others just to make it through the day myself, so there didn't seem to be any way that I could properly care for a colony of 60,000 harmless suburban honeybees as well.

But then, much to my surprise, at the beginning of my fourth year of several dozen weekly bee stings, I unexpectedly but officially became a "think-outside-the-box" novice beekeeper. Michael, the patient apitherapist who shows up every Thursday to administer honeybee stings that stretch from the base of my toes to the top of my scalp, unexpectedly inherited several different beehives. After discussing the idea with Ramon, Michael urged me to let him bring one of his "extra colonies" to my house where it could live in my small backyard.

Obviously, this unexpected living, breathing (*Bashert)* gift was **meant to be**, even though I never thought that I would actually be in a position to adopt 60,000 honeybees who needed a new home. Ramon, who has been my kind and caring helper for close to two decades, and who has routinely received eight to ten stings each week from Michael right after I get mine, loved the idea of having our own home-based supply of honeybees. As a little boy, he had lived with his beekeeping grandmother in Guatemala's *Montanas Pazarajmaja*, so he was enthusiastic about—and right at home with—the idea of caring for several thousand hard-working honeybees.

Michael assured me that it would take only slightly more than a few attentive hours per month of Ramon's time for our transplanted *Apis mellifera* to feel right at home. Plus, he promised that the flowers and trees in my yard (as well as in our entire neighborhood) would benefit and thrive as never before.

As usual, Michael, was right…

***

For the past four years, I've been conducting an informal survey about what I used to refer to as "Celebrity Beekeepers." During that time, I was surprised at how many famous and accomplished people through the ages have gravitated towards sharing their space with these tiny miracle workers. Several of my honeybee-expert friends feel that it's cheating to call yourself a beekeeper if (as the rich and famous often do) you pay someone else to care for and manage your hives. Others feel that any action that makes people more aware of how astonishing *Apis mellifera* are, deserves gratitude instead of criticism.

Below is an abbreviated list of accomplished individuals—both past and present—who share my infatuation with these unique and amazing insects.

ARISTOTLE: This famous Greek philosopher (384 B.C.-322 B.C.) wrote extensively about bees in his most famous work *Historia, Animalium,* and did so from the perspective of a beekeeper.

DAVID BECKHAM: This British Soccer legend has homes in Miami and Los Angeles, but keeps his beehives at his Cotswolds estate in the UK. His wife, *Spice Girl* Victoria Beckham, posted a video of him working with his honeybees on Instagram, and it has been viewed over two million times (so far).

SOPHIA BUSH: Currently living in Bologna, Italy, and working as an educator and the podcast host of *A Work in Progress,* this honeybee advocate has close to four million Instagram followers. In addition to publicizing and supporting a wide variety of bee-friendly organizations, this Global Ambassador for girls keeps two active beehives on her property.

KING CHARLES III: The former Prince of Wales has been keeping bees at his Highgrove Estate in Gloucestershire for decades. His mother, QUEEN ELIZABETH II, also maintained beehives in the gardens at Buckingham Palace in London.

LEONARDO DI CAPRIO: The Academy Award-winning actor was introduced to beekeeping by his mother's boyfriend, David Ward, as a way to de-stress during the Hollywood awards season. Di Caprio has even built his own wooden beehives, which he keeps at his Los Angeles home.

THOMAS EDISON: The famous phonograph inventor (1847-1931) was rumored to dislike the smell and taste of most foods so much that his meals were prepared in an outdoor kitchen. Edison did, however, appreciate the unique qualities of beeswax and honeycomb; he kept his 150 hives (many of which were made of clay and straw) at his Seminole Lodge Florida property.

WILL FERRELL: The actor's property in Laurel Canyon supplies his forging bees with plenty of nectar from Acacia and Oak trees; the result is a rose-tinted honey that his fans purchase from the Flamingo Estate website. The proceeds are then passed along to Cancer for College, which is to his chosen charity. This organization awards scholarships to cancer survivors.

FLEA: For close to a decade, the bassist of the *Red Hot Chili Peppers* has been keeping about 40 hives with almost a quarter of a million honeybees on his Los Angeles property for close to a decade. He refers to them, collectively, as "Flea's Bees."

HENRY FONDA: He may have won an Academy Award for his role in *On Golden Pond*, but his real passion was for the thousands of bees that lived at his Bel-Air estate. Fonda (1905-1982) and his wife gave gift-wrapped honey from "Hank's Bel-Air Hive" to friends and co-workers. His son, Peter, portrayed a beekeeper in the 1997 movie *Ulee's Gold*, and his daughter, activist and Academy Award-winning actress Jane Fonda, starred in the hit Netflix series *Grace and Frankie*.

POPE BENEDICT XVI: An Italian agricultural group gave the Pontiff eight beehives, which now live on the 50-acre papal villa in Castel Gandolfo. Currently, the over 500,000 bees (officially under the care of Pope Francis) produce 600 pounds of honey each year.

MORGAN FREEMAN: The Academy Award-winning actor keeps over a million honeybees in 26 hives on his 124-acre ranch in Charleston, Mississippi. He has become so "one with the bees" that he doesn't even wear protective clothing while working with them.

SIR EDMUND HILLARY: In 1953, Hillary (1919-2008) became the first man to reach the summit of Mount Everest. But before that achievement, he had been a commercial beekeeper at his father's honey farm in Tuakau, New Zealand, which had 1,400 beehives. He often told interviewers that the care and discipline that beekeeping required was what had conditioned him mentally and physically for the rigors of mountain climbing.

SHERLOCK HOLMES: This fictional character—created by Sir Arthur Conan Doyle (1859–1930)—eventually "retired," and devoted his last years to beekeeping. In Laurie King's 1994 novel *(The Beekeeper's Apprentice),* she turned the fictional detective into a mentor for a young apprentice—a female beekeeper named Mary Russell.

JENNIFER GARNER: The star of Apple+'s series *The Last thing He Told Me,* began keeping bees after her daughter was inspired by a book about beekeeping. She and her three children keep their two hives in their Los Angeles backyard, she has described this family-friendly hobby as being "Super fun. It's like a living science experiment."

LEBRON JAMES: The basketball star and his wife, Savannah, have hives that rely on Southern California wildflowers as well as Chinese Elm and Eucalyptus trees. His honey is sold through The Flamingo Estate website https://flamingoestate.com/pages/the-estate, and the proceeds go to the LeBron James Family Foundation, as well as to Everytown for Gun Safety.

SCARLETT JOHANSSON: While working with Samuel L. Jackson on a movie, she expressed her concern about the dangers that bees—and the environment—were facing. During those conversations, the two actors discovered their shared love of bees, which is why Jackson then gave her a hive (including everything she needed to become a beekeeper) as a wedding gift when she married Ryan Reynolds in 2008.

DAYMOND JOHN: The billionaire FUBU star of *Shark Tank* was so inspired by Oregon beekeeper Matt Reed (who appeared on the TV program in hopes of investment interest for his Bee Thinking business) that he set up 30 hives on his property in Dutchess, New York. He now has over a million honeybees, and is very active in the pro-pollinator movement.

JON BON JOVI: The popular musician has a seven acre spread in New Jersey where he keeps enough honeybees to (in the past) qualify for an state-funded agricultural tax exemption. Ever since 1964, New Jersey residents who own more than five acres of land, and have generated more than $500 in agricultural revenue received financial incentives. Thanks to his full-time beekeeper and his honeybees, Bon Jovi's agricultural tax bill was only $104.

TIFFANY HADDISH: Her Central Los Angeles hives are nourished by her sweet potato, thyme, and trumpet flower plants. The revenue from the sale of her honey (available at The Flamingo Estate website https://flamingoestate.com/pages/the-estate) goes to the non-profit She Ready, which helps support Foster Children.

DEBBIE HARRY: The vocalist for "Blondie" is so committed to honeybee welfare that in 2017, the New Wave punk band's eleventh studio album (*Pollinator*) was named to motivate her fans to protect *Apis mellifera*. She keeps beehives at her homes in Connecticut and New Jersey, and is often seen wearing bee-themed hats. Information about her "BEE Connected" campaign can be found on the Blondie website. When she appeared on the Tonight Show with Jimmy Fallon in 2022, she gave him a gift of honey from her own hives.

GREGOR MENDEL: Known as the "Father of Genetics," this monk (1822-1884) was an avid beekeeper and his bee house (at the Augustinian Abby in Brno, Czech Republic) is still in use today. He maintained 50 hives, and was an avid researcher regarding the genetic qualities of different types of bees.

JAMES MIDDLETON: The younger brother of England's extremely popular Princess of Wales (her husband is Prince William), James Middleton discovered beekeeping in 2011 when he was 24 years old. His parents and sisters (Katherine and Pippa) bought him 1,000 honeybees, which he described as *"...the most fantastic birthday gift imaginable."*

JULIANNE MOORE: Combining politics with a love for *Apis mellifera*, this Academy Award-winning actress has made a point of publicly casting her election day ballot at the Burt's Bees voting booth at Merchants' Gate in Manhattan's Columbus circle. Her hives are located in Montauk, New York, and her bees harvest nectar from Asters, Blueberry and Goldenrod plants.

MICHELLE OBAMA: The former First Lady may not have actually worked as a hands-on beekeeper, but in 2009 she and the White House chef (Sam Kass) asked a member of the carpentry staff (Charlie Brandts, who was also a beekeeper) to construct and install a beehive next to her organic garden. Soon afterwards, Brandts became the official White House beekeeper.

KAREN PENCE: In June 2017, Mike Pence's wife installed a beehive at the Vice President's official residence. Before she and her husband left the Governor's residence in Indianapolis, Indiana, she had been a vocal *Apis mellifera* advocate, and promoted August 18th as National Bee Day. She gave CNN exclusive rights to film her first D.C. honey harvest; afterwards, two-ounce jars of her honey were then labeled 'Vice President's Bees,' and given as gifts to visitors.

SYLVIA PLATH: Inspired by her father, Otto, who was a beekeeper as well as a global expert on bumblebees, this American poet was living—unhappily—in Devon, England, when she became a beekeeper. Plath (1932-1962) wrote a number of poems about bees before she committed suicide.

AGNES BADEN-POWELL: The younger sister of the man who founded The Boy Scouts—Lord Robert Baden-Powell (1857-1941)—her bees produced prize-winning honey, and she even kept a functioning hive **inside** her home. In 1910, Agnes Baden-Powell (1858-1945) founded The Girl Scouts movement in England.

ED SHEERAN: He has sold over 150 million records, and at his 16-acre estate in Suffolk, England, his country lifestyle includes chickens, goats, a greenhouse and (of course) bees. One of Sheeran's goals is for his farmland to become ecologically self-sustaining.

MARTHA STEWART: Ever since the 1970s, she has maintained beehives on her properties. She credits the bees with helping pollinate her flower gardens and fruit trees. Stewart also hosts this informative link, https://www.marthastewart.com/8138495/beekeepin

<u>g-for-beginners</u>. She employs a professional beekeeper to manage all of her hives,

STING: Gordon Sumner is the front man for *The Police,* but he became known as Sting because he so often wore black and yellow striped sweaters. He and his wife, Trudie Stylar, have an 86-acre 400-year-old Italian villa in Tuscany, where their bees make honey from the chestnut grove on the property. Sting is also a patron of the non-profit *Bees for Development*, which encourages beekeeping to combat poverty.

PAUL THEROUX: The award-winning author of *The Mosquito Coast* owned over 700 acres of land in Hawaii named *Oceana Ranch*, where he has maintained over 80 beehives. In the past, Theroux (1942-2019) disagreed with Professor Randolph Menzel of the Free University in Berlin, Germany, who claims that honeybees sleep at night, and are not always busy. He always insisted that his *...Bees never stop working.*

LEO TOLSTOY: The famous Russian author of *War and Peace,* Tolstoy (1828-1910) kept so many honeybees at his Russian home that his wife, Sonja, grew tired of seeing him crouched in front of his hives with a protective net over his face. In her diary, she wrote, *"The apiary has become the center of the world for him now, and everybody has to be interested exclusively in bees!"*

MARIA VON TRAPP: After leaving Austria and moving to the US in 1939, *The Sound Of Music* heroine (1905-1987) settled on a farm in Vermont

(The Trapp Family Lodge) where the family's honey was sold. Her husband, George, was the person who encouraged her to become an active beekeeper.

STEVE VAL: Famous for his work with Frank Zappa and David Lee Roth, he keeps bees on his two-acre property in Encino, California. He built the hive supers himself, and after he harvests his honey it's labeled *Fire Garden Honey,* which he refuses to sell but gives as gifts.

Two other high achievers who deserve special acknowledgment for their bee-friendly efforts are:

RICHARD CHRISTIANSEN: In 2015, the Australian founder of the ad agency Chandelier Creative bought a crumbling seven-acre estate in Eagle Rock, a community on the east side of Los Angeles. When he was a child, his family had bees, and after he moved to LA, he installed beehives for several of his well-known friends. The year after purchasing the neglected overgrown, and run-down acreage in Eagle Rock, he established beehives on his nearby Highland Park property. He now sells 19-ounce bottled honey that is sourced from a variety of well-known celebrity beekeepers for $250. All the proceeds from the honey sales go to the hive-owners' chosen charity.

ANGELINA JOLIE: Her involvement with bee issues is closely tied to a UNESCO-Guerlain program that trains women to become beekeepers and honey sellers, while simultaneously helping the environment. The French cosmetic firm has contributed $2 million towards helping 50 female beekeepers in over two dozen global designated biosphere reserves. The goal is to build 80,000 beehives by 2025, which could house as many as 4 billion honeybees.

So far, the program has included women from Bulgaria, Cambodia, China, Ethiopia, France, Russia, Rwanda, and Slovenia. Jolie will be one of the first ten women to be trained as a certified beekeeper. To publicize World Bee Day on May 20, 2021, Jolie posed with her entire naked torso covered with honeybees.

***

When I was a little girl, I was only called "Cry Baby" once. Why? Because I grew up with an inpatient mother in a small family that had many (many) rules. Whenever I was punished—and this usually included different degrees of physical discomfort—if I shed tears, I would be told "*If you want to cry, I'll give you something to cry about.*" In other words, during my childhood, tears (for any reason) were STRONGLY discouraged...

So, by the time I was an adult, I'd trained myself to (1) cry as rarely as possible, and (2) if tears couldn't be avoided, shed them in private rather than in front of other people. To this day, as a septuagenarian, there are probably fewer than a dozen individuals on this planet who have ever seen me really cry. I share this information not as a form of *braggadocio*, but (instead) as an attempted explanation of what one aspect of my pre-Multiple Sclerosis personality was like.

After MS began robbing my body of its ability to follow my mental directives, my tear ducts began to more than make up for lost time. The reason why I'm writing about tears at this point in my honeybee book is that—as happens so very often—another emotionally-tender MS-related event recently saddened me in a particularly unusual way.

I was working on this chapter at the precise time when the beautiful actress Selma Blair began performing on *Dancing with the Stars*. I had taken a special interest in her life story after watching the documentary *Introducing Selma Blair* and reading her memoir (*Mean Baby*). I learned that she had been diagnosed with MS in 2018, and had undergone a grueling stem cell transplant in Chicago. For those of us whose bodies have been negatively affected (or, like me, paralyzed) by this cruel disease, it was astonishing to see her—after only about 1,000 days following her procedure—dance on national television. She even did cartwheels (!) as well as the splits (!).

My girlfriends and I were spellbound as we watched her first two brilliant performances; we loudly cheered her on with the enthusiasm of fraternity boys in front of a televised Collegiate football game. Then, sadly, only three weeks into the competition, Selma's doctors advised her to withdraw from the show because the program's rigorous rehearsal requirements might have triggered hairline stress fractures, among other physical complications.

For those of us who fervently hoped that Selma Blair would win the program's Mirrorball Trophy, and be for MS what Michael J. Fox is for Parkinson's Disease (i.e., a high-profile advocate, figurehead, and fundraiser), it was a demoralizing and sad disappointment. When I watched her final, bittersweet but elegant performance, I don't mind admitting that I cried like a heartbroken teenager.

Over the years, I've interviewed and socialized with countless celebrities, but I've never managed to meet the inspiring Selma Blair. Now, on my ever-growing bucket list, I've added the dream that one of these days I'll be able to meet her in person, and thank her for being brave enough to place her delicate and chronic illness-challenged body on national display. I have no idea if she has an interest in beekeeping or not, but I can guarantee that those of us burdened with MS consider her our hero for being so honest and open. She has shown the world how Multiple Sclerosis has the cruel ability to painfully alter our lives—whether we are celebrities or unknowns—in the most poignant ways.

WHAT THE HONEYBEES TAUGHT ME

- Having several thousand honeybees in my backyard gave me a different perspective about what constitutes a positive relationship between species. My honeybees remind me that Paulo Coelho, who wrote the cherished best-seller *The Alchemist,* knew what he was talking about when he said: *"Friendship isn't a big thing—it's a million little things."*

- In today's America, it's hard not to be "People Magazine" celebrity obsessed. But in a beehive, there's only one celebrity—the Queen—and the other 60,000 honeybees exhibit no envy of her elevated statis. Instead, they happily exist in an interdependent democracy where each and every creature is important and valuable in her own special and ever-changing way.
- Wherever *Apis mellifera* happens to call home—an abandoned barn, a Beverly Hills backyard, a rock formation, or a royal castle—she works with the exact same skill and enthusiasm. Honeybees don't really need humans to "supervise" or "teach" them what to do. We don't need to alter their centuries-old diet or lifestyle. As Thomas Bertram Lance (1931-2013), who was part of the Jimmy Carter Administration, suggested *"If it ain't broke, don't fix it."*
- I love the fact that—when it comes to productivity—the honeybees don't care where or for whom they are working. They are wise enough to follow their own inner schedule, and rely on their own definition and judgment when it comes to "priorities."
- Perhaps one of the reasons that celebrities and performers identify so closely with honeybees is that they also embrace the concept of more than just a single creative identity (i.e., actor and painter, actress and director, musician and author, screenwriter and producer, singer and dancer, etc.). The evolving and multi-talented honeybee cannot be contained or restricted to only one life-long profession. Evidently, the same truism can also be applied to A-listers.

Chapter 15
Honeybees and Death

Death be not proud...
Thou art slave to fate, chance, kings, and desperate
men,
And dost with poison, war, and sickness dwell
John Donne (1572-1631)

It's never easy to talk about death. There is an almost indefinable sorrow and pain that touches every aspect of your life when the Grim Reaper steals someone you love. While I'm not an expert about the technical mechanics of grief, I have lost an unfair number of cherished and remarkable people who were dear to my heart: Both my parents, a charismatic sweetheart, a charming British ex-spouse, three publishers, two editors, my beloved husband, as well as a veritable platoon of very special friends. As any bereaved person will attest, each death etches a painful and indelible scar on our psyche.

When I began to learn about the honeybees' unfeeling attitude toward death, I was genuinely surprised. As humans, we are in close touch with our sources of affection, our emotions, and the need to mourn when we suffer a loss. Our favorite four-winged pollinators, on the other hand, have no room in their tiny bodies for sentimentality. In fact, as anyone who has watched televised episodes of *Castle* or *The Mentalist* might recognize, *Apis mellifera* could easily be categorized as cold-blooded murderers who view death as nothing more than just another physiological domestic task.

I first became aware of this brutal honeybee behavior when I learned about how the hive's incumbent Queen (if able) will try to attack and kill each potential successor as she emerges from her capped royal beeswax cell. But, in Laurie R. King's novel about Sherlock Holmes and his young protégé (*The Beekeeper's Apprentice*), he describes this furious encounter between the potential unhatched developing Queen, and the existing one as an "*angry*" noise. Sherlock explains to his acolyte that "*The lust for murder is not a rational thing. In Queens, it is an instinctual response.*" If the Queen, however, is unable to prevent a young rival from emerging, once the usurper does appear, the result will still be—literally—a fight till the death.

The next example of bloodthirsty bee behavior happens when colder weather arrives, and the colony essentially executes (via expulsion) the hive's drones. Most hives contain one Queen, about 50,000 sterile female worker bees, and as many as several hundred to several thousand drones. Every colony is in a state of continual reproduction, and the required gestation period differs for each type of larva: Queens develop within 16 days, worker bees take 21 days, and the drones require 24 days.

***

During Spring and Summer, the worker bees dutifully care for and nurture the drones because the males are an essential part of the hive mentality. Without available drones, a virgin Queen can neither be impregnated nor fulfill her all-important essential egg-laying duties. Throughout the year, the (increasingly resented) drones are housed and fed and cared for by the females, but other than inseminating a new Queen, the drones contribute zero, zip, *nada*—nothing—to the wellbeing of the finely-tuned machinery that allows the hive to keep functioning and stay productive.

When the virgin Queen takes her "nuptial flight," she may mate with as many as a dozen drones in all. But the mechanics of their lovemaking are nothing less than gruesome. The drone uses his first four legs to grab the Queen in mid-flight, and uses his last set of legs to make sure she cannot escape. Then, he has to reconfigure the position of his abdomen in order to be able to push his penis into her sting chamber. When he ejaculates, it is so powerful that it actually makes a noise. Then, his genitals literally snap off, and he drops to his death.

As soon as cold weather arrives, less nectar is available, which means that the colony's food supply (i.e., honey) gradually shrinks. That's when the annoyed worker bees literally drive the previously pampered drones out from the hive; as a result they are doomed. The prolific Flemish writer Maurice Maeterlinck (1862–1949) described this *Apis mellifera* annual mass murder process in his 1901 book *The Life of the Bee* (which is still in print today), with these words: *"...the stern workers...only recognize nature's harsh and profound laws. The wings of the wretched creatures are torn, their antennae bitten, [and] segments of their legs wrenched off."* Drones that do not die immediately try in vain to reenter the hive, but the worker bees continue to rip at their already damaged wings and legs until they are all dead. When more nectar is available, new drone larvae will be deposited within the colony to keep the circle of *Apis mellifera* life on track.

The often grizzly "groupthink" that dominates the honeybees' unemotional approach to life—plus their sense of survival above all—also applies to any form of disability or illness within the hive or nest. There is no sense whatsoever of either "lending a helping hand" or assisting a family member in need. Why? Because any hint or sign of weakness or vulnerability is interpreted as a direct threat to the rest of the colony population.

The third version of brutal bee behavior happens whenever a Queen (who can live 40 times long than a worker bee) begins to age, or starts to lay fewer eggs. This drop in productivity is referred to as "sputtering," and it spells doom for the ailing Queen, because the entire colony is now potentially at risk. Instead of organized productivity, the atmosphere within the hive becomes frantic, chaotic, and unpredictable.

As her pheromones change, the worker bees begin to realize that their colony is in danger, and a new Queen must be installed as quickly as possible.

Every hive or nest includes potential new Queen larvae that are constantly gestating, and when one emerges, the ailing or elderly Queen is sometimes also attacked by hundreds of her daughters. They surround her body, and use their wings to generate enough heat to kill her in a deadly process that is referred to by beekeepers as "balling."

***

Since I am a person who has lived with a challenging disability for close to half my lifetime, the concept of enforced euthanasia by a mob is both distasteful and frightening. If—like me—you happen to be dependent on others to help you navigate from one day to the next, the idea that your "worth" is inconsequential or that you could be regarded as nothing more than a "burden" is terrifying. I prefer to persistently believe that, as humans, our empathy gene spurs us to be kind rather than cruel. I'm understandably uncomfortable with the Darwinian idea that those of us who have limitations deserve to be eliminated or expelled.

During my past four wheelchair-dependent decades, I've wasted plenty of hours worrying about the potentially annoying impact my disability has on other people—especially the kind souls that I count on to help me as I try to live a meaningful and productive life. As a society, when it comes to those who need our help, most of us try to do our very best to lessen the suffering of others. Individuals who refuse to imagine themselves in such an unwelcome predicament are simply labeled cruel, uncaring, unkind, or unwilling to follow The Golden Rule; *Do unto others as you would have them do unto you.*

***

My first real-life exposure to death definitely broke my heart. I was a 19-year old college student when my father died, and I still think of and miss him every single day. A lifelong Camel smoker, he had been suffering from ill health (asthma, emphysema, and lung cancer) for several years, but young naïve me always believed (thanks to my youthful Stubborn Optimism) that he would get better.

Instead, his health steadily went downhill, and soon I received a sudden flurry of urgent and alarming phone calls from a cousin regarding his decline. A disbelieving and numb version of myself took an evening flight to get home; upon arrival, I went directly to the hospital, where I found my father in a coma, and my mother asleep on a cot in his room. Simultaneously frightened as well as confused, I had no idea of what I was supposed to do.

The kind nurse at St. Mary's Hospital explained that my exhausted mother hadn't left his room for days. In a quiet voice, she suggested that I sit on the bed, hold his hand, and talk to him for as long as I wanted. "Hearing," she kindly told me, "is the last sense that we lose. I'm sure he would love to listen to your voice."

So, for several hours, as my mother slept on the other side of the room, I sat and softly told him about my French classes, my UCLA classmates, and how much I missed seeing and talking to him every day. The hospital was eerily quiet so late at night, and when his breathing changed dramatically I truly didn't know what it signified. Part of me was frozen, and part of me was panicked; I raced to the hallway, yelled for help, and told the nurse that my father was having trouble breathing.

Within a minute or two of us arriving back at his bedside, daddy's struggle stopped completely— and life as I had known it ended. At that precise moment, in an unusual twist of fate, my mother jerked awake, and called out his name. There was nothing I could do except walk over to her cot, put my arms around her tiny frame, and whisper, "Oh, Mama, Daddy is dead."

In the more than 50 years since that awful night, it feels as if death has stolen way too many people who were important to me. But nothing has ever affected me as profoundly as losing (and witnessing the passing of) the very first person who loved me fiercely, unconditionally, and without reserve.

***

One aspect of a honeybee's approach to death is particularly complicated. An angry worker bee can only use her stinger once because there are tiny barbs on her venom delivery system that cause her internal organs to be stretched and destroyed once she attacks. Her lifespan is only about 45 short days, but employing her stinger against a hive intruder or a human being is essentially an unfortunate form of suicide.

In spite of *Apis mellifera's* practical and unemotional behavior when it comes to the demise of other honeybees, there is a long-standing belief among beekeepers that a hive must be informed if there has been a death in its human family. This official notification is designed to prevent the honeybees' demise or departure. This tradition is an important part of a long-standing European and American bee folklore that is known as "Telling the Bees." It revolves around the traditional belief that verbally sharing news whenever an important family event has occurred is essential.

As with anything regarding honeybees, there are countless different versions of how and why this questionable superstition began. Many bee aficionados contend that it began with the old Celtic belief that honeybees know or sense whenever a soul leaves a body. Long ago, in 1858, a Quaker poet named John Greenleaf Whittier (1807-1892) wrote about a recently widowed husband who watches the farm's "chore-girl" as she shares the sad news with the family's honeybees:

"For I knew she was telling the bees of one
Gone on the journey we must all go!
And the song she was singing ever since

In my ear sounds on—
"Stay at home, pretty bees, fly not hence!

Mistress Mary is dead and gone!"

Traditionally, the beekeeper knocks on a wooden wall of the hive, informs the bees out loud about the death, and then places black fabric on top of the hive. Customarily, in 19th century New England, the eldest son would also slightly rotate the beehives in a process called "ricking," which is considered a physical way of acknowledging the major change that had taken place in the family.

In some Eastern European cultures, the news must be delivered to the beehives through a poem or a rhyming song. Part of the old folklore is that failing to inform the bees about a death in the family is essentially an invitation for bad luck to arrive, which could result in the bees either leaving in a swarm or simply dying mysteriously. Many traditionalists also believe that honeybees do not like noisy or hostile environments, and that angry feuds or loud arguments—just like an "unshared" death—will also cause the bees to abandon their hives.

Dated folklore beliefs can be found wherever bees live; in Germany, for example, beekeepers have been known to sing to their apiaries to generate increased honey production. And as long ago as 1750, William Ellis (1794-1872) of Hertfordshire, England, wrote in his book *Modern Husbandman* about the importance of truly loving your bees; otherwise, they will sting you if you don't genuinely like them. A number of beekeepers have told me that their bees can also tell if a person is afraid or angry or anxious, which is why beekeepers strive to always remain calm and quiet whenever they visit their hives.

As recently as 1961, *Folklore* (the Folklore Society's official journal) reported an inexplicable case in which swarms of bees converged on the flower-covered coffin of a much-loved beekeeper who was being buried in a graveyard that was over a mile away from their hives.

It's difficult to know how or why honeybees can be so unfeeling when it comes to death within their own species, but so sensitive when it comes to deceased human beings. There are plenty of beekeepers who prefer to follow the "tell" tradition and be on the safe side rather than risk losing their hives. This mentality was definitely on display when Queen Elizabeth II (1926-2022) died. John Chappel (the beekeeper at Buckingham Palace) placed bows made of black ribbons on Her Majesty's hives before he notified them—out loud—of her death.

***

When my father died, I was a teenager who felt—like most young people do—that even though I'd suffered a horrible loss, life would progress on a never-ending upward trajectory. Within my youthful mindset, I mistakenly believed that the misfortunes experienced by other (i.e., older) people would never come my way because I would be capable and wise enough to avoid the pitfalls that had sabotaged others. Obviously, I was too young to be familiar with the Yiddish expression *"Der Mensch Tracht, Un Gott*

Lacht," which means *"Man plans and God laughs."* Back then, it honestly (truly) never occurred to me that my future life could (or would) hold so many unforeseen stressful—even downright terrifying—developments.

Two of the most devastating life-altering events I was forced to unwillingly experience included divorce and disability, which arrived accompanied by what felt like a freight train full of adjacent pain. By the time I'd turned 50, life had taught me the difference between being merely disappointed and feeling literally overwhelmed by negative life events.

But nothing that came my way shook my entire world the way the death of my sweet husband did. For over 20 years, we had shared the most unlikely of partnerships. I had never known—much less dated—anyone like Tony, and he had definitely not known (or been involved with) anyone like me. We had both been wounded (emotionally and physically) in different ways, which is probably why finding each other when we did, turned out to be such an unexpected miracle for both of us. There were over a hundred guests at our wedding, and I'm sure that many of them secretly thought: *"Well, that is never going to work..."*

It probably surprised everyone—including Tony and me—that our time together turned out to be the happiest two decades of each of our lives. Somehow, miraculously, we were effortlessly able to give each other exactly what was needed for us to finally enjoy some much-longed for healing and nurturing. For starters, how many able-bodied good-looking men would want to love or care for a disabled paralyzed woman in a wheelchair? And how many men would continue to pursue a twice-divorced woman who had blithely turned down several of his heartfelt marriage proposals?

Tony was definitely not a perfect man, but he was exactly the right person for me at precisely the right time. Initially, I had been drawn to him because he was the kindest man I'd ever met, and I loved the way he cared for (and about) his elderly mother—who was also in a wheelchair. There were a number of people in my life who didn't like either of my first two outwardly successful husbands. But all (literally 100%) of my *uber*-protective friends made no secret of the fact that they thought Tony was wonderful. He was that rare human: A creative, empathic, sensitive man whose ego was under control and whose testosterone wasn't the least bit toxic.

Before MS entered my life, my limited romantic history had felt like an out-of-control emotional roller coaster. To paraphrase Shakespeare's (1564-1616) *Othello*, I was "...*one who loved not wisely but too well*." Fortunately, unlike the better-educated, highly-accomplished, multi-lingual, prosperous, and sometimes cruel men I'd loved before, during our decades together, Tony—literally—never (ever) criticized me in any way. Throughout our marriage, I couldn't help but feel that I had somehow acquired an emotional Golden Ticket that allowed me to finally embrace who I was (and what I needed) without fear of annoying, disappointing, or irritating the man I loved.

Nora Ephron once wrote that the secret to [a good] life was to marry an Italian, and I wholeheartedly agree. For his part, Tony made no secret of the fact that—in spite of all the seriously unpleasant complications that can accompany caring for a person with an "incurable, progressive, neurological disease" he wasn't going to let MS ruin our happiness. During our years together, he somehow treated my (extremely challenging) illness the way someone else might consider misplacing one's eyeglasses or forgetting to pick up a needed item at the grocery store: Mildly annoying and challenging, but not anything that could be considered a catastrophic or overwhelming problem.

I fondly remember overhearing a conversation (at one of our annual Christmas parties) that Tony was having with an old friend—the gifted German piano tuner who maintained his treasured Steinway baby grand. The two Chopin super fans were casually talking about the latest huge payout for the Mega Millions Sweepstakes, and Tony said, "*I never bother buying lottery tickets anymore because I won the jackpot when Marilyn and I got married.*" What wife (disabled or otherwise) wouldn't want to overhear her husband say those words? Lucky, lucky me…

But, as history has taught us, "*Every love story is a tragedy if you wait long enough.*" Sadly, a little more than 700 days before my bee venom experiment began, that sad observation proved to be true. The Cliff's Notes version is that after an almost imperceptible decline in energy and wellbeing, which those of us close to Tony wrongly assumed was little more than a subtle sign of aging (he was 78), my sweetheart was diagnosed with Stage 4 Lung Cancer. All that really needs to be said about the following months was that they were unspeakably horrific. Without going into distasteful details, the bottom line is that watching "your person" suffer, struggle, and slowly slip away from you is painful beyond belief.

There were two totally different things about 2017 that kept me afloat. One was the fact that the last thing Tony said to me before he slipped into a coma was "*I love you,*" and the other was that my diverse army of devoted friends worked overtime to nurture, support, and care for me. Still, it took several years for me to get my tear ducts totally under control, and emerge from a persistent fog of confusion, fear, and grief. As a widow, I don't mind admitting that living without Tony is far more challenging than I could have ever imagined.

When COVID-19 struck and the skyrocketing number of deaths continued to grow, all I could think of was the mountain of grief that millions of people who had lost loved ones must be experiencing. Until my husband died, I had been unforgivably oblivious to the overwhelming pain that accompanies losing the special someone who had once been your favorite person on the planet...

WHAT THE HONEYBEES TAUGHT ME

- Few (if any) of us would want to adopt the lack of sentimentality that *Apis mellifera* exhibits when it

244

comes to the deceased. To us, their cold-blooded reaction to a sibling's death is a reminder that (for us, at least) loss can take many forms, and perhaps there is no right or wrong way to adapt to the passing of those we love.

- The lack of drama that surrounds honeybees and death reminded me of what C.S. Lewis (1898-1963) once wrote regarding death: *"There are far, far better things ahead than any we leave behind."*

- I was amazed at how clinical and objective honeybees could be when it came to "weeding out" their siblings or replacing an ailing Queen who was, after all, their mother. As someone who knows more than I would like to about grief, I prefer Anne Lamott's take on loss: *"You will lose someone you can't live without, and your heart will be badly broken, and the bad news is that you never completely get over the loss of your beloved. But that is also the good news. They live forever in your broken heart that doesn't seal back up. And you come through."*

- Honeybees have been spared all the emotional complications of grief and sorrow that we experience. But the succinct lesson I take from that unwanted experience is the reminder—as Queen Elizabeth II often observed—*"Grief is the price we pay for loving."* And I don't think any of us who have known the joys of loving and being loved would have it any other way.

- While the honeybees and their keepers have an accepted "folklore protocol" for dealing with death, human mortality is far more complicated. The fact that we rarely know precisely how to act or exactly what to say when someone dies just means that we are emotionally imperfect human beings.

Chapter 16
Beauty and the Bees

Vanity is the healthiest thing in life.
Karl Lagerfeld (1933-2019)

Like many American women, I've always had a complicated relationship when it comes to the topic of beauty.

Growing up, I envied my lucky friends (like Patsy and Joy) whose moms derived undiluted pleasure from their daughters' appearance. I longed in vain to be fussed over and told that I was pretty, but my mother was a no-frills, strict woman who believed that vanity was ridiculous at best, and that aesthetics, in general, were a waste of time. For as long as I can remember I have always— inexplicably—been visually obsessed with a topic (beauty) that others might consider shallow or superficial. The bottom line is that I have been endlessly fascinated by appearances: My own, everyone else's, as well as any and all items in the world at large.

I was adopted when I was four years old, and the chasm between my youthful desire for beauty and my mother's disdain for anything other than bare-boned cleanliness and practicality insured that our relationship—especially when it came to vanity— would be a conflicted, complicated, and contentious one.

According to family legend, long before I came into her life, my mother (1905-1974) had enjoyed an enviable life as a well-dressed and dance-crazy flapper. During the Roaring Twenties, she and my father spent their whirlwind courtship perfecting the Black Bottom, the Charleston, and other "racy" dances of that era. My mother once told me that during those carefree years, she had owned a cherished and extensive wardrobe of short silk dresses with matching fabric-covered size 4½ dancing shoes.

My parents married in October of 1929, and they were on their honeymoon when the Stock Market crashed, and the Great Depression arrived. Eventually, like millions of other Americans, they had their young dreams shattered and their hearts broken when their money (as well as their families') seemed to evaporate overnight. Later, on top of that grim financial scenario, they also endured the deaths of their two toddlers, who died from diseases (Diphtheria and Scarlet Fever) that no longer pose a threat in today's America. My mother—the once-carefree, plump, and stylishly-dressed flapper—was plunged into a deep depression, followed by a serious health crisis of her own, which ultimately culminated in a sudden as well as dramatic weight loss.

Part of the conflicting soundtrack of my 1950s childhood was my mother's rare (but still surprising) lament that her face, which had once been youthful and line-free, was now covered in unsightly wrinkles. Unfortunately, those were the days long before affordable facelifts were available, laser treatments existed, or retinol skin creams had become ubiquitous.

She would occasionally try a new skin treatment that promised rejuvenating results, but the bottom line was that—for the rest of her life—nothing could diminish her wrinkles. The lines and creases served as a painful visual reminder of the difficult times, and the sorrow that she had experienced decades earlier. Essentially, the hurtful and unfortunate events she'd experienced years earlier stole her youthfulness, and soured her on life.

As a little girl, I longed for my mother's approval. But I soon learned that while she continually supervised my actions, attitudes, and behavior, she was relatively disinterested when it came to my appearance. As long as my clothes were freshly laundered, properly ironed, and my hair was clean and combed, she was satisfied. On the rare occasions when I would be brave enough to ask her if I was pretty, her terse (and annoyed) answer was always, *"Pretty is as pretty does."* In fact, the **only** compliment I remember ever receiving from her about the way I looked was when she commented that my high school graduation photo was "nice."

And the singular motherly piece of wisdom she ever offered when it came to beauty was a terse, *"You'd better stay out of the sun or your face is going to be as full of wrinkles as mine is."*

***

It took me a long time to follow my mother's advice about avoiding the sun's UVA rays, but other than a brief teenage flirtation with seeking a suntan (it was, after all, the era of The Beach Boys), I've managed to escape having any type of serious skin issues. But by the time I was in high school, I noticed that none of my other friends cared nearly as much about their complexions or skincare routines as I did. Avoiding wrinkles had become an unacknowledged but very real priority in my young life.

I clearly remember, as a 14-year-old sophomore, sitting in the school library during study hall (when I should have been doing my homework), and reading the current (circa 1964) issue of TIME magazine. It contained an article about a groundbreaking study conducted at Stanford University in which researchers were looking for links between smoking and women's complexions. To their surprise, they discovered that cigarettes had no visible negative effects on facial skin until menopause hit. But once hormone levels dropped, however, the unfortunate women who smoked had dramatically more wrinkles than their nicotine-free peers of the same age. As you can imagine, after reading that short article, there was no way my lips would ever get near a cigarette. (My mother, on the other hand smoked until she died of a heart attack at 65; I was 24.)

Eventually, I realized that I had somehow made a mental connection between my mother's chronic unhappiness and the visible wrinkles that covered her face. The same way that some people attach special meaning to what money signifies (i.e., freedom, power, and status), I associated facial wrinkles with a basketful of negatives (i.e., anger, disappointment, and sadness).

Today, unlike in my youth, I know a wealth of information about skincare. But it (literally) took me half a century for me to begin learning about the honeybees' unparalleled international contribution to beauty, and the skin-care products that have helped women look (and feel) their best.

***

If you are looking for beauty aids that include hive products, the most unusual name you might encounter is *"Hydroxypropyltrimonium Honey,"* which is primarily used in shampoos and hair conditioners. **Propolis** (sometimes called Bee glue because of its antifungal and anti-seborrheic quality) can often be found in shampoos designed to treat dandruff. And when used in toothpaste, propolis has been proven to measurably reduce dental plaque; it has also been touted for its anti-aging effects when used in facial creams. **Royal Jelly** is believed to stimulate fibroblasts of collogen because of its ability to retain water, and **Pollen**'s high flavonoid content helps seal and strengthens the capillaries that nourish facial skin. Over time, it can regenerate, moisturize, and condition skin cells.

In the beauty business, **Beeswax** is "harvested" by removing the honey, melting the wax, and then filtering out impurities with the help of electric, steam, or solar extractors. Beeswax is often the base for both creams and lipsticks because of its lubricating qualities. As an emulsifying agent, it can be used as an effective stiffener that provides elasticity as well as plasticity. Because it contains B-carotene, it is easily converted into vitamin A, which is an essential component of retinol.

Are you a GOOP follower? If so, you may have seen Gwyneth Paltrow use **Bee Venom** as a milder and more "natural" form of Botox. It has also been used to treat alopecia, atopic dermatitis, psoriasis, and to counteract the visible effects of aging. Researchers at the Kyung Hee University Skin Biotechnology Center in South Korea have determined that bee venom can actually increase collagen formation, diminish circumference, depth and number of facial wrinkles, as well as inhibit photoaging. Who could ask for anything more?

In light of what I have already written about a worker bee's ability to sting only once, this would be a good time to explain that savvy beekeepers have found a safe way to harvest venom without harming the honeybees. By using a flat (impermeable) surface and a gentle electrical current, the confused bees react to the static, but their stingers are not damaged. That way, after they deposit what we want (or need) they— no worse for the wear—are able to return to their hives and resume their other worker bee duties.

***

During the 1960s, the only beauty treatments a teenaged girl like me could rely on were Bonne Bell 10-0-6 Lotion and Noxzema skin cream. I stuck with those two affordable drug store products all the way through college, but when I was 24, my kind and beautiful friend, Toni Sherman, introduced me to a whole new—dramatically more affordable, effective, and expensive—approach to skin care.

In the 1950s, Dr. Erno Laszlo (1897-1973), created elegant and effective soaps, makeup, powders, and creams, that were considered the Rolls Royce of innovative beauty products. He was a Hungarian-born dermatologist who, back in 1927, opened his first skin institute in Budapest. Laszlo rose to fame when he helped Princess Stephanie of Belgium recover from a chronic case of acute acne. Soon, he was treating numerous other royals, as well as a variety of wealthy high-profile patients.

Against the backdrop of Hitler's European aggression, in 1939 Dr. Lazlo moved to New York City, where he opened an exclusive skin institute on Fifth Avenue and became even more famous. The star-studded celebrities who trusted him with their high-voltage skin care needs included the Duchess of Windsor, Marjorie Merriweather Post, Grace Kelly, Katharine Hepburn, Marilyn Monroe, Jacqueline Kennedy, Audrey Hepburn, as well as Cecil Beaton and even Cary Grant. He soon developed his own line of skin care products, which was eventually purchased and produced by Chesbrough-Ponds.

By the time I was 24 years old, my wrinkle phobia had already been in full swing for over a decade, so I followed my wise and generous friend's advice, and became a fervent proponent of Laszlo's unorthodox brilliance. At the time, his unique water-based approach was considered both controversial and revolutionary. Unlike other cosmetic icons of that era (i.e., Elizabeth Arden, Estee Lauder, Merle Norman, etc.), Laszlo concluded that wrinkles develop when skin is flaccid or lax. This can occur for a variety of reasons, including sun damage and sudden weight loss. Facial skin can also sag when too much heavy foundation or thick moisturizer has been applied too often. He was of the opinion that in order to maintain a youthful complexion, pores needed to be small rather than stretched, and skin needed to be buffed and taut.

Back then, Laszlo's expensive products were only sold in top-tier department stores such as Bergdorf Goodman or Saks Fifth Avenue. Juggling my miniscule "mad money" budget in order to keep my required supply of his beauty products up to date became my number one vanity-centric indulgence. I would literally scrimp and save when it came to the purchase of shoes, haircare, clothes and even (gasp!) books, in order to keep my bathroom medicine cabinet well-stocked with the required large cotton balls, as well as the half-dozen costly products needed to religiously follow the Hungarian dermatologist's strict protocol.

I was able to follow his twice-a-day routine for the next eleven years, but one of my most serious MS challenges occurred when I was no longer able to control or use my right arm, hand, or fingers. Since consecutively splashing one's face 30 times in a row with soapy water —morning and night—was part of the required Lazlo regimen, there was no way I could continue with the use of only my (not particularly reliable) left hand. So, for the next two decades, I scrambled to find an effective alternative disability-friendly skin care solution.

In the Spring of 2011, when Kate Middleton married Prince William, I read several articles about a number of British Royals who had prepared for the all-important wedding festivities by indulging in under-the-radar Bee Venom Facials. Like Erno Laszlo products, these topical treatments were very controversial, pricey, and they also required finding a qualified bee-savvy aesthetician.

Of course, at that point in my life—long after I was no longer the Health and Fitness Editor—there was no way I could afford a $350 facial. Eventually, however, after several weeks of sleuthing on Amazon, I learned about a company in New Zealand that sold a facial cream that contained small doses of actual Bee Venom. Much to my delight, when the cream arrived, I could tell that it would make a worthy (and much more affordable) replacement for my much-missed Erno Laszlo obsession.

Fast forward to 2019, and the start of my weekly sting sessions. Before long, I learned that my favorite Ukrainian professor not only had over 100 beehives, but he also sold honey, as well as a variety of auxiliary *Apis mellifera* products including— Hallelujah!—tiny vials of locally-sourced freshly-harvested Bee Venom! I was practically speechless when he casually confided to me that he was a consultant for the New Zealand cosmetics company that manufactured the bee venom cream that I'd been faithfully using for the past eight years!

***

If and when you begin using skincare products that have been created with the help of honeybees, you'll be joining millions of other past and present beauty-conscious females throughout history. Here's a short list of renowned *Apis mellifera* fans who have used bee products as part of their customized beauty regimen:

• Nefertiti (1370 BC–1330 BC) was the glamorous wife of the Egyptian Pharaoh Akhenaten
• Cleopatra (69 BC-30 BC) the legendary beauty-obsessed daughter of Ptolemy was married four times (including to Mark Antony), and was also the mistress of Julius Caesar
• Poppaea Sabina (30-65 AD) was Nero's second wife, and reportedly used a facial lotion made of honey and milk seven times a day.
• The women of China's Ming Dynasty (1368-1644) used a mixture of honey and ground orange seeds on their faces to eliminate blemishes, and give their skin a youthful glow.
• In England, Sarah, Duchess of Marlborough (1660-1744) was the subject of my UCLA senior thesis. During her era, she was considered "vain" because she created and used her own secret beauty elixir, which was made from diluted honey.

• Queen Anne of England and Scotland (1665-1714) used a honey and oil mixture to beautify her hair.
• Madame du Barry (1743-1793) was Louis XV's last mistress, and she routinely used a face mask made of honey to enhance her complexion.
• A cave painting that is about 15,000 years old (from the *Cueve de la Arana* in Spain) shows a woman gathering honey.

***

According to the Mintel Group Ltd. (a global privately-owned market research firm), 75% of today's consumers are "interested" in purchasing a skincare product that includes honey. In order to satisfy that growing demand, as many as 60% of new cosmetics may include bee products, botanical, or herbal ingredients. The company also estimates that the use of naturally-derived skincare products will soon generate over $180 billion in sales. And as part of this growing trend, 75% of beauty product consumers are likely to use cosmetics that contain hive components during the next decade.

I'm not sure if these bee beauty products estimates are correct or not, but one bee-savvy woman told me recently that it can take up to ten thousand worker bee stings to harvest just one gram (0.35 ounce) of usable bee venom. Considering how many domestic and international firms are selling skin care items that include bee products, our treasured honeybees will definitely be working harder than ever in the years to come.

If I listed every small startup or large conglomerate that used bee venom or honey or pollen or propolis in their products, I would probably have to write an additional 67,000-word volume in order to be accurate and inclusive. I can, however, give you a tiny glimpse of what is currently happening in the glamorous world of cosmetics and skin care. Here are a few randomly-selected companies that may or may not have already become a crucial part of your own *Apis mellifera* beauty consciousness:

Domestic

In **California**, the powerhouse skincare line Eighth Day was founded in 2009 by Dr. Antony Nakhla, a dermatologist and reconstructive surgeon who has a special interest in skin cancer. He discovered that Manuka honey can dramatically help skin tissue regenerate, and includes it in his cosmetic serum. Also based in "The Golden State" is Mary Louise Cosmetics. Akilah Mary Louise Releford, now CEO, started a bee-centric skin care firm in her dorm room at Howard University. The company is currently located in Los Angeles.

In **Georgia**, The Savannah Bee Company has been creating bee-dependent and bee-friendly products for the past two decades. In addition to offering soothing creams and balms, they also sell their own raw honey. Their Bee Cause Projects has provided hundreds of grants to schools as a way to help students learn more about the vital role that *Apis mellifera* plays in all of our lives.

Anthony Maxfield, Gwen Maxfield, and Christina Sirlin realized—back in 1998—that honey and beeswax had "astonishing and rejuvenating properties". Since then, the **Hawaii**-based firm Honey Girl has even expanded to the increasingly popular Chinese market.

Burt's Bees has been innovatively using bee products since the early 1980s. The company was founded in **Maine** by a former New York photojournalist who became a beekeeper, and a cosmetics-savvy artist from San Francisco. According to legend, Roxanne Quimby (who had a good head for business), asked Burt Shavitz to teach her about beekeeping, and she soon decided to create bee-centric cosmetics. Their famous lip balm was launched in 1991, and the company(now located in Durham, **North Carolina**) currently sells over 150 different products.

Barbara Chappuis, RN, developed the Bee Naturals skin care line to heal her hands, which were dry and chapped as a result of washing them so often at the hospital where she worked. Located in **Missouri**, her company now offers a variety of balms, creams and lotions designed to therapeutically heal and nourish stressed-out skin.

Beeline Skin Care is a small **New Hampshire** company that was created when its founder, a chemist named Susan Lanphear, developed work-related skin issues. Since she couldn't find any existing products that weren't irritating, she developed her own line that relied heavily on both beeswax and honey.

Claire Marin is a **New Yorker** who uses honey from the Catskills as part of her Catskill Provisions firm, which creates beauty, food, and drinks designed to improve overall well-being. Bees are even working their way into the fragrance market with Ellis Brooklyn Bee Eau De Parfum in **New York**.

Another American company (headquartered in Seattle, **Washington**) got its start back in 1986, when two strangers met at a Chicago diner. Since then, the company and its "Egyptian Magic All-Purpose Skin Cream" has become a cult favorite among celebrities. It's clientele list believes in the unparalleled efficiency of honey-based beauty products.

International

Bee U Organics in British Columbia**, Canada**, has become a popular and respected bee-friendly cosmetics firm.

In London, **England,** the beauty and wellness company Mahoni focuses on products that feature Manuka honey, which only comes from New Zealand and Australia. When you order a bee product wrap from Great British Products in Gloucestershire, a packet of flower seeds is included to help bees pollinate outdoor plants and retrieve nectar. And Liz Earle Beauty, which was founded by a popular author and beauty expert, began in the Isle of Wight.

Guerlain, the **French** cosmetics powerhouse, is currently offering an "Abeille Royale Advanced Youth Watery Oil," which is a 95% natural serum that includes French Black Bee honey, as well as royal jelly. These *Apis mellifera* ingredients have been shown to be particularly effective at moisturizing and repairing skin. Additionally, Sisley-Paris—an independent French luxury cosmetic, skin care, hair care, and perfume company—sells a pricey sleeping mask that is made using organic raw thyme honey and turmeric.

The high-end **German** company Augustinus Bader, actually imports and includes Lindon honey from Bulgaria in its hand lotion. And in Milan, **Italy**, the Wonder Company has created a variety of bee-based beauty products.

The Dr. Hauschka Company has maintained bee colonies in a biodynamic herb garden in Eckwalden, **Germany** since the 1980s, and relies on beeswax for many of its skincare products.

The **Netherlands**-based company Gisou uses raw honey in all of its products to enhance treatments from skin care to hair health. The company was founded by Negin Mirsalehi, whose Iranian family had been beekeepers for over five generations. Even though the company was only established in 2015, it has quickly become an international powerhouse in the health and beauty field; in the US, Gisou's products are available at Sephora.

South Korea has a robust reputation for high-quality skincare, and Bombee Honey Company is a particularly popular firm, as are both Savor Beauty and Superegg.

The **Swedish** company SJO has a loyal following for its Happy Honey Facemasks, and **New Zealand's** Manuka Doctor Skincare line has thousands of international customers.

Since 1921, the **Swiss** company Weleda has been famous for using the finest natural and organic ingredients. Their Body Butter is an essential part of their home-grown NATRUE skincare line, which relies on beeswax.

WHAT THE HONEYBEES TAUGHT ME

- Women in Egypt had already discovered the beauty potential of beeswax and honey thousands of years ago, long before vanity (and the changing post-World War I-era standards) had turned the cosmetics industry into a major economic influence.

- A number of beekeepers insist that the best way to improve a complexion is to **eat** honey every single day rather than applying it topically. As I've noted before, however, there is never a shortage of differing opinions about what is or isn't "true" when it comes to bees and their byproducts.

- In light of how many billions of dollars—and millions of millions of *Apis mellifera* contributions—who is to say for sure whether or not "*Beauty is only skin deep*"?

- In 2019, my favorite Ukrainian professor and beekeeper taught me how to create my own (affordable) skin cream and serum by mixing bee venom and Methylene Blue with an FDA-approved coconut oil and vitamin E delivery system. With the help of my indispensable assistant, Ramon, I make a fresh batch each month, and we mix all the ingredients in my small kitchen. I like to think that my Blue Bee Beauty cream is an accessible, affordable, and worthy substitute for Erno Lazlo's products.

- Years ago, MS decided to take my right arm as a hostage. Previously, however, my morning beauty protocol—before showing up at the *Los Angeles Times* building each day—was relatively time-consuming. First, there was the five-step Erno Laszlo system, then there was blush, eyeliner, mascara, and lipstick. But for the last several decades, my morning routine is a quick five-minute cleanse, mini-exfoliation, and a thin layer of my homemade face cream. I no longer use foundation, blush or powder; and my complexion (according to people who have known me for decades) has never looked better. The only extra touch is a light layer of lipstick. It took me half a lifetime to learn what German-American architect Ludwig Mies van der Rohe (1886-1969) meant when he declared that *"Less is more."*

Chapter 17
My Personal Protocol

A person can get used to almost anything given enough time—personality will grow around adversity the way tree roots will grow around a rock, shaping itself in response to the immovable.

HOW I LEARNED THE ART OF SEDUCTION
Malisa Febos

Four years ago, when I started this book, I had no idea how it would end. But now, after thousands (and thousands) of honeybee stings, I'm sure that while this particular volume may be finished, my bee venom-MS journey will continue to gradually evolve; even if it does so baby step by baby step.

There's no way I could ever erase the horrific memory of the terror I felt when, on a cold December morning in London, a Harley Street neurologist—examined my MRI results, and warned me that—"With an incurable degenerative progressive neurological disease" like mine—the expected lifespan was 20 years from the date of diagnosis. At the time, I was 38 years old and, for the next decade, I lived with an invisible stopwatch superglued to my psyche. My Stubborn Optimism struggled as it fought with my fear level; I couldn't stop wondering how many (or how few) future birthdays or Christmases might lay ahead.

The good news is that my stint as Health and Fitness Editor (during those long-ago *Los Angeles Times* years) had taught me that MDs were not inherently infallible, and that medical "miracles" happened every day. Obviously, it simply went against every fiber of my being to accept—without a fierce struggle—such a dire diagnosis.

My one huge regret is that I was so frightened about the mere **possibility** of MS that I grabbed at every potentially credible explanation for my body's rebellious state, which was a regrettably inept stalling technique. Maybe my problem was due to a pinched nerve...or a dietary imbalance... or too much stress...or...

But after the MRI revealed the presence of those honest-to-God much-dreaded brain-tissue lesions, I did a rapid attitudinal 180-degree reassessment. And ever since that awful moment of truth, I have worked overtime as an obsessed health-focused detective/investigator/researcher in hopes of finding anything and everything that might contribute to an alternative life-affirming outcome. This book has been the result of that genuinely rewarding and unorthodox MS solution-seeking journey.

It's important to (again) remember that every case of Multiple Sclerosis is different, and every MS patient is unique. I am happy to share my experiences, but I am also fully aware that just because I had a particular outcome, those results can never be considered universally applicable. The thousands of honeybee stings I experienced (and endured) have not "cured" my MS (of course, I want to add the word "yet"), but they definitely improved both my overall state of mind and my physical well-being.

I am still forced to use a wheelchair to get from point A to point B, and I routinely need to rely on other people to help me (in countless situations and numerous times) each and every day.

But in spite of what able-bodied people would categorize as an absence of progress (due to my continued lack of mobility), those bee-venom Thursday afternoons—a reliable mixture of laughter and pain and pastries—have changed and enhanced my life emotionally, physically, and spiritually. I am particularly grateful that (thanks to the 50 weekly sacrificial stinging honeybees) my once-pervasive and deeply unwelcome aura of depression lifted slowly but steadily, the same way that a fog bank dissipates in the sunshine.

I still suffer from frequent bouts of frustration due to things that I'm not (yet) able to do, but as my health slowly improves, my life now includes fewer and fewer irritating physical limitations. And I'm thrilled to report that I no longer cling to the silly and corrosive belief, which was wrong on so many different levels, that MS is in my life because I had annoyed or offended whoever or whatever might be in charge of The Universe. These days—unlike the ones when I felt like a hopeless victim of a cruel and wicked fate—I simply feel full of gratitude for how incredibly lucky I have been, as well as for how responsive my aging and battered body continues to be.

My favorite sign of honeybee-derived improvement is one that other people would never even be aware of, but to me it is huge. Back in the days when I lived in my little bungalow all by myself, years before I'd even met my future husband, much-missed Tony, my sense of proprioception was severely altered and definitely impaired. As a result, dropping items, knocking things over, or spilling liquid was a continual, embarrassing, and frustrating occurrence—in one annoying form or another.

These days, as I sit in my recliner, I am able to use pretty fabric "throws" in a variety of colors to cover my lap. But before the bee stings began, I was forced to use large, washable, terry cloth beach towels. Why? Because (inevitably) I would drop or spill something, and I needed to have the most absorbent "lap protection" covering I could find. I still cringe when I remember how a well-meaning friend brought me a gift of a very ugly and utilitarian large, black, plastic adult-sized bib, which she felt would (at least) finally protect my clothes from those annoying and reoccurring clumsy accidents.

Now, thanks to the bee stings, those embarrassing days are behind me. And (because my health today is so improved and my body now works so much better) I simply can't remember the last time I spilled something. And, on the rare occasions when I do happen to drop a pen or some papers or the phone or the TV remote control, my much-improved left arm strength and range of motion means that (more often than not), I can retrieve the object in question "all by myself" without having to ask anyone else for help. That's only one small example of how my lengthy honeybee experiment has diminished my MS-induced depression and dependency.

Of course, I still have occasional episodes when I battle being sad or feeling sorry for myself or getting frustrated. But now those harmful negative emotions are truly the exception rather than the rule. Once I could tell that the bee venom had halted the slow-moving downward MS trajectory, my life-long Stubborn Optimism returned with a vengeance. And, as a result, I became reacquainted with my genetic belief in a better tomorrow.

This book was inspired by my gratitude to the tiny female fighters whose last living act continues to remind me that something truly wonderful (i.e., physical improvement) can be triggered by something seriously toxic (i.e., bee venom). I also owe a major debt to my ever-evolving Thursday support group, as well as to the brilliant authors, kind beekeepers, and wise researchers who are invested in the *Apis mellifera's* well-being, and who generously taught me so much. Thanks to them, I was able to be a far more open-minded and patient woman than anyone (including me) could have ever predicted. Those 10,000 bee stings inspired me to (finally) make my own health a top priority, which let me to cast myself as an activist layperson advocate for alternative (as well as ancient) healing modalities.

I am no longer a discouraged and frightened MS patient who is terrified of humiliating and never-ending future losses, increasing levels of disability, as well as constant discomfort. Instead, I've learned to think of my decades-long health struggle as a real-life mystery novel; there's simply no way anyone can accurately predict if or whether my body will ever be able to do the things it once did, or revert to the way it used to be.

I do, however, know for a fact that *Apis mellifera* has forced me to acknowledge that Mother Nature has many astonishing secrets up her sleeves. The tenuous progress that my compromised and confused body has taken over the past four years have—in countless minuscule ways—taught me that Roald Dahl (1916-1990) was right when he wrote "*...and above all, watch with glittering eyes the world around you because the greatest secrets are always hidden in the most unlikely places. Those who don't believe in magic will never find it.*"

Obviously, just like Ted Lasso and his AFC Richmond team, "I **believe**."

***

One of the biggest lessons my MS saga has taught me is that sometimes we have been given childhood beliefs that follow an outdated or faulty road map. In my case, because I was adopted by a couple who was old enough to be my grandparents, I was led to believe that I was the healthiest individual residing on Planet Earth. Both my parents were smokers who—by the time I joined their household—had experienced a variety of physical ailments that seemed to increase with each passing year. In retrospect, I can now understand why, from their much-older vantage point, everything about their much-younger little girl—from my boundless energy level to my hearty appetite to my enviable sleep habits—was nothing less than remarkable.

They commented about my "*astonishing good health*" so often that I truly believed them, and gradually became convinced that nothing could or would ever go seriously wrong with me physically. I was sure that the Good Luck Goddesses had supplied my physique with its very own customized Teflon shield. I honestly believed that (physically, at least) I was invincible. For that reason, even though I was deeply interested in and fascinated by the mechanics of good health, the adult me definitely neglected to take good care of my own body.

Unfortunately, the older I got the harder it became (literally and figuratively) to walk the walk. My childish sugar addiction grew with each passing year, and when I should have been focusing on natural, wholesome, nutritious meals, I was (instead) kneading bread or making fudge or baking cookies. When I should have been paying attention to the quality of the meals I ate, the factor that truly influenced my dietary patterns was (tsk, tsk, tsk) the number I saw on the bathroom scale, how snuggly my clothes fit, which size I happened to wear, or what I saw reflected in a full-length mirror.

***

It's common knowledge that as adults the shelf life for blaming our parents ends with our 20s, so this is an explanation rather than an indictment. My mother was a petite Kentucky-born housewife who served simple meals that centered around her favorite foods, which (unfortunately for me) happened to be vegetables. From mustard greens to okra to cauliflower and spinach, every dinnertime inevitably included items that I found truly distasteful. Since there would be tension and disapproval if I didn't "clean my plate," I became adept at moving things around, eating items that I actively disliked, and getting through each meal with the knowledge that— eventually—there would always (Halleluiah!) be dessert once the vegetables were removed from the table.

This unfortunate dinnertime dessert dynamic helped solidify my conviction that food (instead of being regarded as health-promoting fuel for the body) could be exclusively viewed as an emotional treat or a reward. Obviously, I am solely responsible for not being sensible enough to outgrow this juvenile mindset, and I have paid dearly for my nutritional childishness.

Thanks to my mother's no-nonsense meals, however, and the fact that I grew up with few sodas or snacks and no processed or fast foods, I actually did enjoy a very healthy childhood. But once I became an adult, and no longer had to eat those dreaded vegetables, things got a lot trickier. When the stresses of being a grown-up hit me with full force (i.e., lengthy family dramas, motherhood, divorce, demanding work situations etc.) taking care of myself became the last and much-neglected item on my lengthy to-do list.

When life simply became too difficult (e.g., a broken heart, an angry editor, financial problems, whatever) instead of adding healthier foods or nutritional supplements to my lifestyle, I chose the easiest (and most familiar) alternative. Since my stomach was already in knots, I tried to soothe my emotions by literally living off of my dangerous and nutrient-deficient version of "comfort food."

For a very (very) long time, whenever hunger pangs paid a visit, I would simply exist on three empty-calorie items: strong black coffee, a variety of chocolate or cookies, and heavily-buttered popcorn. With the benefit of perfect hindsight, I can see what an awful recipe for disaster I created for myself. The result of such a reckless and ridiculous lifestyle was that my immune system and my microbiome were so depleted that I became the perfect candidate for a horrific autoimmune disease, and the ideal repository for MS.

***

A number of professional health practitioners have been baffled by how long I have fought to rebuild and regain my health. In one of her interviews, actress Selma Blair summarized the elusive mystery that is MS by commenting that this sort of autoimmune disease is simply the outward manifestation of a really really unhealthy (i.e., gunked up) body. And while I may not be as impatient about my quest for recovery as others are, I am often baffled by the amazing amount of "cleansing repair work" that it has taken to achieve such small improvements. I can't help but wonder how one formerly "*astonishingly healthy*" body can require so much attention, time, effort, and restorative TLC to just get back on track, and function the way it was meant to.

If I had an emotional and physiological crystal ball, it would reveal that I flip-flop between being (on good days) a cheerful Pollyanna and (on days when I can't blow my nose or am unable to turn a page) a Debbie Downer. That's when the dark forces whisper, *"What you are doing is simply too little too late,"*

Back in 1978, when I was inundated with scary single-mother issues, I hung a small plaque near my kitchen sink so I would be sure to see it every single day. President Calvin Coolidge's (1872-1933) wise words inspired and motivated me then, and they still do;

"Nothing in the world can take the place of persistence. Talent will not; nothing is more common than unsuccessful [people] with talent. Genius will not; unrewarded genius is almost a proverb. Education will not; the world is full of educated derelicts. Persistence and determination alone are omnipotent…"

***

273

Below is my very personal list of some of the potentially health-enhancing tools that have helped me during my unorthodox journey:

BVT: For the past four years I have been receiving approximately (sometimes fewer, sometimes more) 50 bee stings administered by Michael, my much-admired local apitherapist. He arrives each Thursday during his lunch hour, and then proceeds to use his lengthy metal tweezers and live bees to sting me—from the base of my toes to the top of my head—along acupuncture points. The goal is to boost my immune system, as well as provide antibacterial, antiviral, and anti-inflammatory benefits to my sluggish, toxic, uncooperative body. Applying ice to the specific area that will receive a sting helps diminish the pain somewhat, but the honest truth is that (to varying degrees) every sting still hurts. Obviously, I would rather have the ten minutes of pain from each sting than the continuing functional decline that is part of the official definition of MS.

Beverages: On TV and in the movies, people almost always have a beer, a glass of wine (or something stronger) in their hands. I, on the other hand, rarely have more than six alcoholic drinks during an entire year. Why? Because after I learned how damaging liquor can be to the soft-as-butter brain tissue, I became—for the most part—a teetotaler. Did you know that in the days before EpiPens existed, a person who was severely allergic to bee venom and was experiencing anaphylactic shock, could be "rescued" by ingesting a quick dose of any alcoholic beverage?

When I realized that the beneficial health-promoting effects of bee venom could be immediately neutralized by a drink of wine or rum or vodka or whiskey, that sort of shaken or stirred "buzz" suddenly lost its appeal.

Instead, I rely on healthier beverages. Thanks to what I learned from Dave Asprey's books, I begin each morning with a Bulletproof coffee. (Mix hot black coffee, two scoops of collagen protein powder, and two large spoonful's of butter in a blender for a faux cappuccino.) The rest of the day, I sip of CCF (Cumin, coriander and fennel seeds) or strong green tea.

Every week, when Michael would arrive to administer my bee stings, I couldn't help but notice that while Jeanne would often choose hot chocolate, and I would be enjoying my Bulletproof coffee, Michael always asked for a hot mug of green tea. His discipline inspired me to research the benefits of what many people call "The healthiest beverage on the planet." Green tea's magic bullet is a catechin called *epigallocatechin-3-gallate* (EGCG), which is an antioxidant that reduces the formation of free radicals, and also helps protect cells and molecules.

Additionally, I also paid very close attention to the advice I found in an eye-opening book by Integrative Neurologist Dr. Kulreet Chaudhary. In *The Prime*, she recommends CCF tea, which is a blend of ground coriander, cumin, and fennel seeds. In Ayurvedic medicine, digestion is considered the cornerstone of good health, and this particular blended tea has been used for centuries as a way to help detoxify the body. Dr. Chaudhary also encourages her patients (and readers) to avoid compromising the healthy function of our lymph system by eliminating cold drinks, as well as (boo hoo) ice cream, from our diets.

Food: For some inexplicable reason, I've always preferred reading recipe collection and health books far more than novels. And while I've learned a vast amount of information from them, I've never quite managed to be as disciplined or logical as I should be when it comes to what I eat. The good news is that I'm not really tempted to eat large amounts of animal products, but the bad news is that my extremely dangerous sweet tooth is still alive.

Thanks to Dr. Cate Shanahan's book *Deep Nutrition*, I learned to avoid the eight different dangerous oils that are ever-present in the Standard American Diet: Canola, corn, cottonseed, grapeseed, rice bran, safflower, soy, and sunflower. For a long time, I tried to follow Dr. Joel Furhman's advice from his books *Super Immunity* and *Eat to Live*, but the fact that I'm not crazy about most vegetables made it an uphill battle for me. I've also been a big fan of Dr. David Perlmutter's books (full disclosure—before he retired from his practice in Naples, Florida—I was briefly one of his patients), as well as those by Dr. Mark Hyman, who is the head of functional medicine at The Cleveland Clinic. Intellectually, I know exactly what I **should** eat for optimum health, but—more often than not—emotionally, I just need (and want) a cookie…

The National Multiple Sclerosis Society has recently announced that adhering to The Mediterranean Diet can help those of us with MS avoid developing cognitive (memory and thinking skills) impairment. Essentially, to protect and repair our brain tissue, it's wise to eat lots of fruits and vegetables, as well as fish, nuts, and whole grains. Olive oil is the preferred fat, while baked goods, highly processed foods, and red meat need to be avoided.

Hive Products: Each day, I make it a point to: Use bee venom eye drops, which have allowed me to avoid or postpone cataract surgery for the past five years; take one of the Professor's Royal Jelly capsules; eat a teaspoon of raw organic honeycomb; and—when possible—I indulge in a relaxing session of Bee Air. Each morning, I also use a small amount of my anti-wrinkle bee venom skin cream, and —of course—my sweetener of choice is always the Professor's dark local raw honey.

Hyperbaric Oxygen: After three and a half years of weekly bee stings, I added hyperbaric sessions as a way of self-treating potential (extremely scary) bedsores. Back in 2012, my temporary weekend helper "ghosted" me, which meant that my body didn't get moved from my recliner for over 48 hours. As a result, I developed a bedsore so severe that I was hospitalized for eight days, placed on five different intravenous antibiotics, forced to undergo surgery, and then I contracted MRSA (*Methicillin-resistant Staphylococcus aureus*). A good-sized chunk of my right buttock had to be removed, and ever since then it's been a priority to pay very close attention to the state of the posterior skin that I sit on.

After reading a number of books about hyperbaric oxygen—all of which were written by MDs—I learned how effective HBOT (hyperbaric oxygen treatment) can be when it comes to wound healing. And, believe me, a bedsore is a wound! Pressurized oxygen also has a number of other potential health benefits as well, and it appears to act like a booster shot for whatever additional medical modalities are already part of your own wellness journey. While this can be costly, the good news is that there are hundreds of Restore Hyper Wellness franchises scattered across the country that provide affordable hyperbaric treatments.

Intermittent Fasting: For over a decade, I've tried to go without eating for twelve to 16 hours each day because I was so inspired by Michael Mosely's 2012 BBC documentary about intermittent fasting. After researching the process, I couldn't help but feel that the same way we allow our automobiles and other machinery to experience "down-time," we also need to do the same for our own bodies. Giving our digestive system a rest pays big dividends, and my personal favorite benefit is that intermittent fasting boosts your body's metabolism.

Pain: Every MS patient I know (including yours truly) deals with a rotating version of physical discomfort. For some people, the small muscles next to bone tissue can cause deep pain, and a different type of searing ache can strike the larger muscles as well. In my case, I have endured what feels like rock-hard Charley Horse cramps in my thigh muscles, and sometimes in my right bicep. When you have my level of MS, there is no way you can "shake it off" or "walk it out," so I was happy when a friendly physician suggested that I try (if an Aleve didn't do the trick) Cannabis Infused Gummies.

I may be the only Septuagenarian on the planet who has always vehemently disliked the smell of pot. But I will happily admit that the odor-free gummies literally make my pain disappear within 15 minutes. For me, luckily, the bonus is that they taste like fruit, and there is no "weed odor." If you live in a state that allows medical marijuana products to be sold, my preferred brand is WYLD Elderberry, which has a THC/CBN ratio of 2:1.

Pilates: Even though I am unable to move anything other than my left arm, using the vertical spring mechanism on a Pilates frame provides a great relief for my muscle stiffness, as well as for my torque-related spinal pain. Someone (almost always the indispensable and lovely Ramon) has to first help me get from my wheelchair onto the mat. Then, he puts each leg into the knee and ankle spring loops and moves my legs for me. In another example of how remarkably lucky I have always been, my generous friend Sonia Cooper insisted that I keep "her" Pilates Cadillac frame at my home so that Ramon and I could use it as often as possible. She claims that her apartment is *"Too small for the device,"* but I believe that she knew how beneficial and valuable the assisted-movement and suspended exercises were for my body. With my level of MS stiffness, a half hour session provides the perfect dose of pain relief.

Physical Therapy: No matter what other proactive avenues you choose to follow on your wellness journey, muscle movement needs to be at the very top of your list. One of the bitter truths about MS is: *If you don't move it, you will lose it.* Without exercise, your circulation pathways will transition from a sluggish slow-moving internal system into an immovable network of very stiff and uncooperative muscles. For the past 17 years, I've been receiving physical and occupational therapy for a minimum of two hours a week. And on the rare occasions when I am forced to miss a session, my stiffness and pain levels rise dramatically.

Naturally, being Miss Positivity, I frequently pat myself on the back for being so "disciplined," or at least I did until I interviewed *Superman* actor Christopher Reeve back in 2004. His two strongly-delivered pieces of advice to me were: (1) *Work as hard as you can to stay as healthy as you can, and do it for as long as you can. That way, when science comes up with a cure for those of us who have lost our mobility, we will be poised and ready to immediately benefit from such a discovery.* And (2) *Move as much as possible, even—especially—if other people have to manipulate your limbs for you.* Reeve told me that he had a rotating staff of 18 different people who helped him clock in close to five hours of physiotherapy each and every day in his quest to once again be able to walk.

Supplements: After I read Ana Claudia Domene's amazing book (*Multiple Sclerosis and (lots of) Vitamin D: My Eight-Year Treatment with The Coimbra Protocol for Autoimmune Diseases*) about how Dr. Coimbra from Brazil had discovered a link between autoimmune illnesses and vitamin D deficiencies, I began taking several thousand units of this nutrient each day.

Also, several decades ago, when I still had frequent UTIs and unwelcome bouts of urinary urgency, my friend Fritz Bell taught me about Low Dose Naltroxone, which had been used by Dr. Bernard Bihari, a Harvard Medical School graduate, to help MS patients. For me, it made a world of difference, and on outings with my husband or with friends, I was able to stop worrying about where the nearest handicap-accessible restroom might be.

Body Work: I am (as usual) extraordinarily lucky when it comes to being the recipient of excellent health-advancing advice. A brilliant (and kind) clinical massage therapist, Dale G. Alexander, Ph.D., M.A., L.M.T., has taken a particular interest in my struggle to cope with (and potentially conquer) M.S. He frequently (and kindly and skillfully) uses a block of time after our Thursday bee stings to work on my hijacked muscles.

For the average patient, however, one-on-one body work can be a huge financial burden. If you cannot afford regular sessions with a qualified licensed massage therapist, the next best option is to get your hands on a Theragun. This hand-held device really helps sore, tired, and uncooperative muscles.

Twenty minutes with this costly (but worth every penny) self-massager pays enormous dividends. It literally puts the competition to shame, and has improved both my circulation and my muscle tone.

***

Yikes! After reading the above self-care categories, I realize that this *bon voyage* summary, has turned into the longest chapter of the book! Seeing—in black and white—just how costly, intimidating, and time consuming it can be to battle MS (if you chose to avoid pharmaceuticals, as I have done). Rebuilding your immune system and reclaiming your health can morph into a rather demanding and full-time occupation. But when this disease challenges every aspect of your life and takes control of your body, the bitter truth is that you simply don't have any other effective or workable alternatives.

The above information has not been offered as a prescription, but merely as a glimpse into how I have coped—through several decades—with my particular multiple sclerosis challenges. My wish is that you will be able to carve your own helpful and very personal battle plan as you travel towards a healthy, productive, and pain-free future.

May your tomorrows be ones in which MS is little more than an ever-shrinking shadow over your life's inspiring legacy.

WHAT THE HONEYBEES TAUGHT ME

- While I've downplayed the pain factor, bee stings (obviously) hurt. And as each honeybee gives me her final gift of venom, I remind myself that the discomfort I feel might be the price I'm paying today for not taking better care of myself (diet, lifestyle, stress level, etc.) when I was younger, and mistakenly thought that my body was invincible.

- It's no secret that I have always been a very impatient person, but the honeybees have taught me the value of learning how to wait (even if I do it impatiently). For most of my life, I've collected turtle figurines because I always loved the Aesop's fable *The Tortoise and the Hare*. Who could have predicted that my lengthy BVT experiment could potentially turn into a slowly-learned 21st century zen lesson.

- Thanks to my study of the honeybee world, I stumbled upon this quote by Hungarian Nobel Laurate Albert Szent-Gyorgyi (1893-1986) who wrote, *"Improving diet and exercise and removing toxins and stressors from the home and workplace have a profound and lasting effect on the prevention and treatment of the majority of modern chronic diseases."* Talk about Food For Thought!

- Having MS for so long has taught me that it's important to not let it overtake every aspect of your life. I exert a good chunk of energy each day to make sure that my clothes are attractive, and that my lifestyle is as close to the pre-MS me as humanly possible. Doing so is never easy, but I know—thanks to Henry David Thoreau (1817-1862)—that clinging to your ideal self-image is essential. To keep me on track, I have his brilliant quote within my line of vision in several different rooms: *"Go confidently in the direction of your dreams! Live the life you have imagined."*

- I (like most people) used to be afraid of a bee sting, but in a 180° change, I've learned to welcome what I once feared. Since then, I've been able to apply this attitude reversal to an ever-growing number of other beliefs and opinions that once seemed cast in stone.

Acknowledgments

For my part, I am almost contented just now, and very thankful. Gratitude is a divine emotion: It fills the heart, but not to bursting; it warms it, but not to fever.

Charlotte Bronte (1816-1855)

No writer is able to truly work independently. But a one-handed author like me is far more indebted to the world at large than most. Every single person in my enchanted *Apis mellifera* world has helped (in big ways and in small) shoulder the burden of creating this book.

Without the extraordinary generosity of Jeanne Hunter, Tom Safran, Toni Sherman, Arnold Shapiro, Donna Brown Agins (whose beautiful artwork is on the cover), Penelope Queen, and Courtney Sherman, none of these pages could or would have ever been written. For decades, they have propped me up, and refused to let me fall no matter how grim life's circumstances happened to feel. There is no way that I can ever repay the kindnesses they have shown me over the past 50 years.

A small army of typists have struggled with trying to translate my illegible handwriting, mold their schedules around mine, and follow my erratic thought patterns as I continually flipped from one chapter, paragraph, and sentence to another. Profound thanks for their energy, enthusiasm, and patience. These overworked, underpaid, and unsung angels include: Joseph Maroney, Danyale Miller, my cherished teenaged typist Clare Ringle, and Elizabeth Turchen. Special thanks to Adrian Hersh, who became my favorite Austin, Texas remote-control IT genius. All of their fingers deserve a long luxurious vacation.

Thanks also to my ensemble of "California girl" supporters: Karen Bayless, Mia Ciminella, Hilary Gauntt, Susanna Janssen, Katie Kinsey, Karen MacKain, Angela Shaw, and Susan Schorr. My Florida "Village" includes: Sonia Cooper, Missy Gannon, Jeanne Hogue, Jeanne Hunter, Jeanne O'Donnell, Anne Rodgers, Rita Romano, Elizabeth Thieman, Elisabeth Tretter, Mimi Vail and Beth Varian. The treasured Ramon Poz also deserves kudos for his countless acts of kindness.

The trio of experts who have tirelessly worked to ensure that my MS-compromised body stays as cooperative as possible include: Dale Alexander, Kelli Jacobs, and Ellen O'Bannon. I know what a challenging patient I can be, and I hope they know how much I rely on their skillful (and talented) hands.

When it comes to family, I've always believed that I hit the jackpot with my two remarkable sons (B.G. and Geoffrey), their fabulous wives (Tori and Susan), and my four perfect grandchildren (Cara, Morgan, Ivy, and Gray). Also, *Mille grazie* to the endlessly supportive and lovely Laura Lynch. Lucky, lucky me…

I have shamelessly picked the brains of every bee-centric and honey-obsessed person I could find, and yet I still feel as if I have only scratched the surface. Blessings to the inspiring (and astonishingly gifted) Michael Szakach, who actually planted the creative-possibility seed that eventually turned into this book. And, of course, the incomparable Professor Vetaley Stashenko, who changed my life forever. My debt of gratitude to this brilliant and unique man can never be repaid.

A special thanks goes to each of the "First Readers" who made sure that this book's grammar, punctuation, and syntax were up to Sister Martha's exacting standards. They all deserve a standing ovation.

And, finally, any and all errors that can be found within this volume are totally my responsibility.

Recommended Reading

I cannot live without books.

Thomas Jefferson (1743-1826)

APIS MELLIFERA

Ashton, Paul; Holmes, Sherlock, *Practical Handbook of Bee Culture*, MX Publishing, (2017)

Asis, Moises, *Abridged Apitherapy: 101 Clinical Forms,* CreateSpace, (2017)

Beck, F. Bodog, M.D., *The Bible of Bee Venom Therapy,* Health Resources Press, Inc., (1997)

Brackney, Susan, *Plan Bee,* Penguin Group (USA) Inc. *(2009)*

Broadhurst, C. Leigh, Ph.D., *User's Guide to Propolis, Royal Jelly, Honey, and   Bee Pollen,* Basic Health Publications, (2005)

Brown, Royden, *How to Live the Millennium: The Bee Pollen Bible,* Plains Corporation, (1989)

Chandler, Philip, *The Barefoot Beekeeper 4th Edition,* Lulu.com, (2014)

Coleman, Mary Louise, *Bees in the Garden and Honey in the Larder,* Doran Doubleday, (1939)

Combs, Dawn, *Sweet Remedies: **Healing Herbal Honeys**,* Story Publishing, (2019)

Cote, Andrew, *Honey and Venom: **Confessions of an Urban Beekeeper**,* Random House, (2020)

Ellis, Hattie, ***Sweetness and Light**,* Three Rivers Press, (2004)

Enders, Paul**, *An Introduction to Apitherapy: When Nothing Else Helps, Try the Power of the Honey Bee**,* BoD, Norderstedt, (2020)

George, Sara, ***The Beekeeper's Pupil**,* Headline Book Publishing, (2002)

Hanson, Thor, *Buzz: **The Nature and Necessity of Bees**,* Hachette Book Group, Inc., (2018)

Hartlib, Samuel, ***A Reformed Commonwealth of Bees**,* Forgotten Books, (2019)

Horn, Tammy, ***Bees in America: How the Honey Bee Shaped a Nation**,* The University of Kentucky, (2005)

Howard Strawbridge, Brigit, ***Dancing with Bees: A Journey Back to Nature**,* Chelsea Green Publishing, (2019)

Hubbell, Sue, ***A Book of Bees**,* Houghton Mifflin Company, (1988)

Hubbell, Sue, ***A Country Year**,* Mariner Books, (1999)

Jarvis, D.C., M.D., ***Folk Medicine**,* Fawcett, (1985)

Jukes, Helen, *A Honeybee Heart Has Five Openings,* Simon & Schuster UK Ltd., (2018)

Kearney, Hilary, *Queen Spotting,* Storey Publishing, (2019)

Kidd, Monk, Sue, *The Secret Life of Bees: A Novel,* Viking Penguin, (2002)

King, R. Laurie, *The Beekeepers Apprentice,* Picador Reading Group, (1994)

Lefteri, Christy, *The Beekeeper of Aleppo,* Penguin Random House, (2019)

Dr. Levitt, Joshua, *Honey Healing Kitchen,* Splash Campaign, (2020)

Dr. Levitt, Joshua, *The Honey Phenomenon: How This Liquid Gold Heals Your Ailing Body,* Splash Campaign, (2015)

Longgood, William, *The Queen Must Die: And Other Affairs of Bees and Men,* Penguin Books Canada Ltd., (1985)

May, Meredith. *The Honey Bus: A Memoir of Loss, Courage and A Girl Saved by Bees,* Thorndike Press, (2019)

McKibben, Bill, *Oil and Honey: The Education of an Unlikely Activist,* Henry Holt and Company, (2013)

Mingo, Jack, *Bees Make the Best Pets,* Conari Press, (2013)

Mortimer, Frank. *Bee People and the Bugs They Love,* Kensington Publishing Corp., (2021)

Mraz, Charles, *Health and the Honeybee,* Queen City Publications, (1995)

Munz, Tania, *The Dancing Bees,* The University of Chicago Press, Ltd., (2016)

Paska, Megan, *The Rooftop Beekeeper: A Scrappy Guide to Keeping Urban Honeybees,* Chronicle Books, (2014)

Petterson, Joachim, *Beekeeping: A Handbook on Honey, Hives & Helping the Bees,* Fog City Press, (2015)

Picoult, Jodi, *Mad Honey,* Ballantine Books, (2022)

Pollan, Michael, *The Botany of Desire,* Random House, Inc., (2001)

Pundyk, Grace, *The Honey Trail: In Pursuit of Liquid Gold and Vanishing Bees,* St. Martin's Press, (2008)

Ransome, M. Hilda, *The Sacred Bee: In Ancient Times and Folklore,* Dover Publications, Inc., (2004)

Root, A.I., *ABC and XYZ of Bee Culture,* Revised Edition, Generic, (1978)

Seeley, D. Thomas, *Honeybee Democracy,* Princeton University Press, (2010)

The Xerces Society, ***100 Plants to Feed the Bees,*** Storey Publishing, (2016)

Ulmer, Mikaila, ***Bee Fearless,*** G.P. Puntam's Sons, (2020)

Wagner, Pat, ***How Well Are You Willing to Bee???,*** Wildes-Spirit Design & Printing, White Plains, MD., (1994)

HEALTH AND WELL-BEING

Asprey, Dave, *The Bulletproof Diet: Lose Up to a Pound a Day,* ***Reclaim Energy and Focus, Upgrade Your Life,*** HarperCollins, (2014)

Asprey, Dave. ***Fast This Way: Burn Fat, Heal Inflammation, and Eat Like the High-Performing Human You Were Meant to Be,*** HarperCollins, (2021)

Asprey, Dave. ***Game Changers: What Leaders, Innovators, and Mavericks Do to Win at Life****,* HarperCollins, (2018)

Asprey, Dave. ***Head Strong****,* HarperCollins, (2017)

Asprey, Dave. ***Super Human: The Bulletproof Plan to Age Backward and Maybe Even Live Forever,*** HarperCollins, (2019)

Attia, Peter, M.D., ***Outlive: The Science & Art of Longevity,*** Harmony Books, (2023)

Blackburn, Elizabeth, PhD. Epel, Elissa, PhD, *The Telomere Effect,* Grand Central Publishing, (2017)

Buettner, Dan, *The Blue Zones Solution: Eating and Living Like the World's Healthiest People,* National Geographic Society, (2015)

Carter, Mildred; Weber, Tammy. *Body Reflexology: Healing at Your Fingertips,* Penguin Group, (1994)

Chaudhary, Kulreet. *The Prime: Prepare and Repair Your Body for Spontaneous Weight Loss,* Harmony, (2016)

Chutkan, Robynne. *The Microbiome Solution: A Radical New Way to Heal Your Body from the Inside Out,* Penguin Random House, (2015)

Collen, Alanna, *10% Human: How Your Body's Microbes Hold the Key to Health and Happiness,* HarperCollins, (2015)

Fuhrman, Joel, M.D., *Eat to Live,* Little, Brown and Company, (2003)

Fuhrman, Joel, M.D., *Nutritarian Handbook: And ANDI Food Scoring Guide,* Gift of Health Press, (2012)

Fuhrman, Joel, M.D., *Super Immunity,* HarperCollins, (2011)

Gundry, Steven R., M.D., *The Plant Paradox: The Hidden Dangers in "Healthy" Foods That Cause Disease and Weight Gain,* HarperCollins, (2017)

Hyman, Mark, M.D., *Young Forever: The Secrets to Living Your Longest, Healthiest Life,* Little, Brown Spark, (2023)

Li, William W., M.D., *Eat to Beat Your Diet: Burn Fat, Heal Your Metabolism, and Live Longer,* Hachette Book Group, Inc., (2023)

Merrell, Woodson, M.D., *The Detox Prescription,* Rodale Inc., (2013)

Moore, Jimmy; Westman, Eric C., M.D., *Keto Clarity: Your Definitive Guide to the Benefits of a Low-Carb, High-Fat Diet,* Victory Belt Publishing, (2014)

Mosley, Michael, M.D.; Spencer, Mimi. *The Fast Diet: Lose Weight, Stay Healthy, and Live Longer with the Simple Secret of Intermittent Fasting,* Atria Books, (2013)

Ni, Maoshing, M.D., *Secrets of Longevity,* Chronicle Books, (2006)

Perlmutter, David, M.D., *Brain Maker: The Power of Gut Microbes to Heal and Protect Your Brain for Life,* Little, Brown Spark, (2015)

Perlmutter, David, M.D., *Drop Acid,* Little, Brown Spark, (2022)

Perlmutter, David, M.D., *The Grain Brain Whole Life Plan,* Little, Brown, and Company, (2016)

Petrucci, Kellyann, M.S., N.D., *Dr. Kellyann's Bone Broth Diet*, Rodale, (2015)

Shanahan, Catherine, M.D.; Luke Shanahan, *Deep Nutrition: Why Your Genes Need Traditional Food,* Flatiron Books, (2018)

Taussig, Rebekah, Sitting Pretty, HarperOne, (2020)

Van Der Kolk, Bessel, M.D., *The Body Keeps the Score: Brain, Mind, and Body In The Healing of Trauma,* Penguin Books, (2014)

Wahls, Terry, M.D., *The Wahls Protocol,* Penguin Group, (2014)

Zinczenko, David; Moore, Peter, *The 8 Hour Diet,* Rodale Inc., (2013)

Recommended Viewing

A picture is worth a thousand words.

Confucius (551 BC-479 BC)

A Bee's Diary, Smithsonian Channel, (2022)

https://www.smithsonianchannel.com/special/a-bees-diary

https://www.imdb.com/title/tt18309322/

Bee Czar, Discovery Channel Series, (2022)

https://www.discovery.com/shows/bee-czar

My Garden of a Thousand Bees, Directed by David Allen, TV Show Series "Nature" S40Ep1, (2021)

https://www.mygardenofathousandbees.com

https://www.pbs.org/wnet/nature/my-garden-thousand-bees-about/26263/

Bees Tales From the Hive, Directed by Wolfgang Thaler and Herbert Habersack, NOVA/WGBH, (2020)

https://www.pbs.org/wgbh/nova/bees/

Keeping the Bees/Kovan, Directed by Eylem Kaftan, (2020, 2019)

https://www.imdb.com/title/tt12285116/

https://www.netflix.com/title/81414893

Tell it to the Bees, Directed by Annabel Jankel (2019)

https://www.imdb.com/title/tt7241926/

How to Bee, Directed by Naomi Mark (2019)

https://www.imdb.com/title/tt7713210/

https://howtobee.ca/watch/

The Pollinators, Directed by Peter Nelson, (2019)

https://www.imdb.com/title/tt10187550/

Honeyland, Keep the Hives Alive Directed by Tamara Kotevska & Ljubomir Stefanov, (2019)

https://www.imdb.com/title/tt8991268/

Keep the Hives Alive, Directed by Trent Waterman, (2016)

https://www.youtube.com/watch?v=2DSODl2vjoQ&t=2s

Hive Alive, Directed by Joanne Stevens, (2014)

https://www.amazon.com/gp/video/detail/B08T4WZ7CF/

Bee People, Directed by David G. Knappe, (2014)

https://www.amazon.com/Bee-People-David-Knappe/dp/B07BZSQ9MG

Why Bees are Disappearing, Marla Spivak, TEDGlobal (2013)

https://www.ted.com/talks/marla_spivak_why_bees_are_disappearing

More than Honey, Directed by Markus Imhoof, Kino International, (2013)

http://www.morethanhoneyfilm.com/see-the-film.html

Queen of the Sun: What Are the Bees Telling Us?, Directed by Taggart Siegel, Collective Eye Films, (2010)

http://www.queenofthesun.com/store/watch-now/

The Strange Disappearance of the Bees/ Le mystère de la disparition des abeilles, Directed by Mark Daniels, (2010)

https://www.imdb.com/title/tt1740679/

Colony, Directed by Carter Gunn and Ross McDonnell, (2009)

https://www.imdb.com/title/tt1480655/

https://www.amazon.com/gp/video/detail/amzn1.dv. gti.96a9f759-e5a7-daeb-caea-b884f35a2d67?ref_=imdbref_tt_wbr_pvt_aiv&tag=imdbtag_tt_wbr_pvt_aiv-20

Vanishing of the Bees, Directed by George Langworthy and Maryam Henein, Hive Mentality Films & Hipfuel Films, (United Kingdom, 2009)

https://www.imdb.com/title/tt1521877/

Who Killed the Honey Bee?, Directed by James Esrkine, (2009)

https://www.imdb.com/title/tt1496043/

https://www.bbc.co.uk/programmes/b00jzjys

The Last Beekeeper, Directed by Jeremy Simmons, (2008)

https://www.imdb.com/title/tt1415238/

The Secret Life of Bees, Directed by Gina Prince-Bythewood, (2008)

https://www.imdb.com/title/tt0416212/

Bees - Living for the Queen, Directed by Wolfgang Thaler & Herbert Habersack, (1998) https://www.amazon.com/Bees-Living-Queen-Wolfgang-Thaler/dp/B00KTL36MO

Ulee's Gold, Directed by Victor Nunez, (1997)

https://www.imdb.com/title/tt0120402/

Bees - Living for the Queen, Directed by Wolfgang Thaler & Herbert Habersack, (1998)

https://www.amazon.com/Bees-Living-Queen-Wolfgang-Thaler/dp/B00KTL36MO

Made in the USA
Columbia, SC
13 November 2023

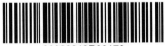

26029319R00170